Defend Your Life II

ALSO BY SUSAN REX RYAN

Silent Inheritance
Defend Your Life

Defend Your Life II

Vitamin D: *Better Health from Preconception through Adulthood*

Susan Rex Ryan

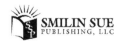
SMILIN SUE
PUBLISHING, LLC

DISCLAIMER

Published in February 2019 by Smilin Sue Publishing, LLC.

smilinsuepublishing.com

ISBN: 978-0-9845720-7-6

Book design by BookWise Designs.

Dedication

To the thousands of members in the Vitamin D Wellness support group.

CONTENTS

INTRODUCTION

Over a decade ago, I began discovering the scientific research about vitamin D's health benefits. As I participated in medical conferences around North America, I understood more and more about this amazing nutrient. As a layperson, I felt an obligation to share my findings in a book called *Defend Your Life*

As *Defend Your Life* was my first book, I had no idea if anyone would read it. But they did; *Defend Your Life* was enjoyed around the world. And the book won an award: the international Mom's Choice Award® for family-friendly creativity.

My knowledge of vitamin D and its partners also culminated in the development of a daily nutrient regimen called the Vitamin D Wellness Protocol.

In turn, I founded the Vitamin D Wellness support group on Facebook. At the time of this writing, the group includes more than 17,000 members. *Defend Your Life II* is dedicated to those members. Membership is on the rise and spans five (six, if anyone living on Antarctica is a member) continents. Every day my team of volunteer administrators and I tackle a variety of members' stories— some about their vitamin D successes, others with good questions.

The content of *Defend Your Life II* addresses a plethora of information about vitamin D and comprises four parts. The first part discusses the basics of vitamin D including its cofactors. The second part addresses the role of vitamin D from preconception through early childhood. Part III contains the latest scientific research about vitamin D lowering the risk of common but serious medical conditions. Finally, the last part spells out the Vitamin D Wellness Protocol so it is easy to understand and follow.

I sincerely hope you will enjoy learning about how vitamin D and its partners may improve your and your family's health-related quality of life.

—*Susan Rex Ryan*

PART I

Vitamin D Overview

1

VITAMIN D BASICS

Dust particles danced in the sunlight, streaming through the windows of a chemistry laboratory at Germany's University of Goettingen. Stepping back from his microscope, Dr. Adolf Otto Reinhold Windaus carefully wiped his delicate, wire-rimmed glasses with a clean, white handkerchief. Leaning his back against the laboratory bench, he thoughtfully pondered his profound discovery: vitamin D!

Dr. Windaus's studies had originally concentrated on complex alcohols known as *sterols*, which led him to research of the chemical structure of *cholesterol*. His cholesterol research subsequently led to his discovery of a chemical called *7-dehydrocholesterol*—the chemical precursor to vitamin D. He also demonstrated that vitamin D is really a steroid that is converted to vitamin D when exposed to sunlight.

In 1928, Dr. Windaus won the Nobel Prize in Chemistry for his work on sterols and their connection to vitamin D. But vitamin D has a history well before the twentieth century.

Since ancient times, we have known about the substance now called vitamin D. For example, Hippocrates, the father of modern medicine, used sunlight exposure to treat a type of tuberculosis.

More than a thousand years later, rickets, a disease characterized by soft and disfigured bones, emerged in Europe. Caused by vitamin D deficiency, this malady was initially documented in England in 1650. During the nineteenth century scientists began understanding the positive effect of ultraviolet B (UVB) sunlight on treating rickets. We discuss vitamin D and its significant connection to sunlight in the next chapter.

Now let's take a look at vitamin D basics. We know that vitamin D is technically a steroid hormone, produced by our bodies when we: expose our skin to UVB light; consume large quantities of fatty fish or vitamin D-fortified foods; or take a vitamin D supplement.

Unless you bask daily in UVB rays under optimal conditions stated in Chapter 2, eat immense amounts of wild-caught fatty fish, or follow the daily Vitamin D Wellness Protocol stated in Chapter 18, you most likely have inadequate levels of vitamin D that may increase your risk of developing an array of medical conditions.

Many people—across generations and geographic locations—suffer from deficient vitamin D levels because their lifestyles do not usually include vitamin-d-rich foods, unprotected sunbathing, or taking the proper supplements.

- A 2017 study published in *The Journal of the American Osteopathic Association* found high, vitamin D deficiency prevalence worldwide. Osteopathic doctors Kim M. Pfotenhauer and Jay H. Shubrook conducted a comprehensive review of vitamin D including its physiology, deficiency risk factors, diagnosis, and treatment. They found that about one billion persons globally, or nearly fifteen percent of the world's population, have a vitamin D level of less than 30 ng/mL, well below the optimal level of 100 ng/mL.

Symptoms of low vitamin D include a host of common complaints such as muscle weakness, fatigue, bone pain, and chronic back pain, as well as susceptibility to contagious illness including the common cold. Vitamin D deficiency is easy to diagnose by a simple blood test (see Chapter 4) and treat by taking up to three over-the-counter supplements daily (see Chapter 18).

Let's understand the basic process of vitamin D in the body. Our health is controlled and maintained by trillions of cells, the smallest units in the human body. The body's organs comprise millions of cells. Cells contain components called receptors that control what vitamins, minerals, hormones, and other substances (medications, free radicals, etc.) can enter or depart a cell.

Vitamin D receptors (VDR) receive and, in some cases, produce activated vitamin D. VDR are present from head to toe: in our brains, eyes, hair follicles, and skin as well as in, inter alia, our cardiovascular, endocrine, gastrointestinal, immune, musculoskeletal, nephrological, neurological, reproductive, and respiratory systems.

The most natural way to obtain vitamin D is from moderate exposure to UVB rays from the sun. When your skin absorbs UVB rays, your body interfaces with a chemical called 7-dehydrocholesterol and produces **initial** vitamin D (cholecalciferol). Alternative sources for vitamin D are cholecalciferol from over-the-counter supplements and limited foods.

It is interesting to note that cholecalciferol is included as an "essential medicine" in the World Health Organization's (WHO) List of Essential Medicines (EML). The EML "contains the medications considered to be the most effective and safe to meet the most important needs in a health system."

Once cholecalciferol is produced in the skin cells, it enters the blood stream and travels to the liver. The liver processes—by hydroxylation—vitamin D into **circulating** vitamin D (calcidiol or 25-hydroxyvitamin D).

Circulating vitamin D travels along two distinct paths. First, the kidneys convert calcidiol into **activated** vitamin D (calcitriol or 1,25-dihydroxyvitamin D3). This activated vitamin D interacts with the parathyroid glands to maintain calcium blood levels.

Second, if circulating vitamin D remains in your bloodstream after calcium levels are maintained, the liver converts the leftover circulating vitamin D into activated vitamin D. The "excess" activated vitamin D travels in the blood to your tissues and cells and attaches to VDRs to perform functions essential to great health:

- Regulate gene expression;
- Reduce inflammation;
- Fight viral and bacterial infections; and
- Regulate cell differentiation, proliferation, and natural death (apoptosis).

These mechanisms of action are vital to protecting you from developing a wide array of medical conditions including autoimmune disorders, cancer, heart disease, and osteoporosis.

How Safe is Vitamin D Supplementation?

Vitamin D toxicity is rare. As you have learned, vitamin D supplementation mimics the production of cholecalciferol in your body when UVB rays strike your skin. Scientific studies indicate that our bodies can naturally absorb about 20,000 IUs from daily exposure to UVB rays to make a sufficient amount of vitamin D to protect us from most illnesses.

Furthermore, a 2019 study in Ohio reported that, after seven years of over 4,700 psychiatric patients supplementing with vitamin D3 either 5,000 or 10,000 IU day, there were no issues with calcium and parathyroid levels. "Due to disease concerns, a few patients agreed" to supplement with 20,000 to 50,000 IU daily! The researchers concluded in the *Journal of Steroid Biochemistry and Molecular Biology* that "long-term supplementation with vitamin D3 in doses ranging from 5,000 to 50,000 IU a day appears to be safe." Therefore, a daily vitamin D supplementation of about

10,000 IU, specified in Chapter 18, is safe for most people.

Please note that persons who suffer from kidney disease, sarcoidosis, or hyperparathyroidism should definitely consult a medical practitioner before taking vitamin D supplements. In addition, folks who are using cardiac glycosides (digoxin) or thiazide diuretics should check with their health care provider prior to using supplemental vitamin D.

Concluding Thoughts

Vitamin D is actually a steroid that is produced when cholecalciferol is in the body. Sources of cholecalciferol are UVB light, a limited number of foods, and over-the-counter supplements. Cholecalciferol is recognized by the WHO as an essential medicine under "Vitamins and Minerals."

Too much vitamin D in the body is rare. Nonetheless, the safest method of controlling your vitamin D supplementation is to monitor your circulating vitamin D and calcium levels at least every six months until you have achieved a vitamin D status that you wish to maintain.

In the next chapter we look into primary sources of vitamin D.

2

SOURCES OF VITAMIN D

The most natural source of vitamin D is exposure from the sun's UVB rays. The sun has provided its light including UVB rays as long as we have inhabited the earth. People originally lived and worked outdoors. They wore little, if any, clothing. And they lived near the equator, the closest distance from the sun.

Fast forward to the Industrial Revolution in the nineteenth century, two twentieth-century world wars, vast technological advances, and global economic markets. Today people live and work indoors. They commute and travel by enclosed conveyances. Air conditioning has become widely used at work places and in homes. These lifestyles have contributed to vitamin D deficiency.

Let's briefly review a decades-old campaign launched by the cosmetic industry. Seeking additional revenue, the cosmetic industry endeavored to market its products as not only beauty but "health" aids. In the 1970s, the cosmetic business reportedly began funding medical schools' dermatology departments with the intent to influence the American Medical Association (AMA) to educate the public about the dangers of sunlight. In 1989, the AMA issued the warning that caused millions to purchase and apply sunscreen and sunblock products. Well, you know the rest. The sunscreen business totals in the billions of U.S. dollars, and the sun scare continues today as does the prevalence of vitamin D deficiency.

Outdoor UVB Light

We do not need to hide our skin from the sun. The body possesses an inherent mechanism to produce just the right amount of vitamin D from the sun. The skin can produce about 20,000 IU of "intake" vitamin D a day depending upon a number of situational factors. After the body acquires enough D (usually about 20 minutes of ideal UVB exposure), the skin's safety mechanism turns off the initial production of vitamin D. Moderate exposure to the sun is healthy.

A number of factors affect the degree of UVB sun rays absorbed by our bodies to produce vitamin D including:

- Geographic location. Location is paramount to making vitamin D in your skin. The closer to the equator (lower latitudes), the higher the altitude, the better opportunity to acquire vitamin D-rich sunlight.

- Time of day. The higher the sun is in the sky, the better to obtain vitamin D from the sun. The hours of 10:00 AM to 2:00 PM are the best times to get vitamin D from direct sunlight. If your shadow is shorter than your height, you are in a potential vitamin D-producing window.

- Season. Many medical studies have demonstrated seasonal effects on vitamin D levels. The sun shines the longest period of time during the summer and the shortest timeframe during the winter.

- Cloud cover. An azure sky is highly preferable to cloud cover. UVB light is decreased by about 50 percent when penetrating cloud cover.

- Air quality. An adverse product of industrial civilization is ozone pollution, which absorbs UVB sun rays before they can reach your skin.

- Age. The older one is, the more challenging it is to obtain and maintain adequate vitamin D levels from sunlight. As people age, the concentration of the vitamin D precursor (7-dehydrocholesterol) in the skin decreases.

- Weight. Overweight and obese people have difficulty producing adequate vitamin D. As vitamin D is fat-soluble, the body's fat cells absorb this essential nutrient, decreasing its availability to the organs, tissues, and cells.

- Skin pigmentation. Melanin, the pigment in your skin, absorbs UVB rays. The darker your skin color, the more difficult it is to make vitamin D in your skin. People with dark skin may require up to 10 times the sun exposure that light-skinned people need to produce vitamin D. African Americans have staggering rates of low vitamin D and accompanying incidences of medical conditions associated with vitamin D deficiency.

- Glass windows. Sunning by a glass window or door may feel soothing but it will not help you make vitamin D. Glass eliminates at least 95 per cent of UVB rays.

- Sunscreen and cosmetics. The marriage of cosmetics and sun protection factors (SPF) will reduce the ability for skin to make vitamin D. The application of either product to your skin most likely will block UVB sunlight.

- Clothing. Not only are we encouraged to "cover up" in the sun but some clothing including swimwear contains SPF chemicals! The more clothing we wear in the sun, the less vitamin D is produced in our skin.

Indoor UVB Light

Optimal conditions for producing vitamin D from the sun are dependent on a number of elements. Some factors we can control, and others we cannot. So, what about using indoor sources of UVB light to produce vitamin D in our skin? For almost a century, UVB lamps have been used to treat medical conditions.

Decades later, tanning beds became popular. People tend to frequent tanning facilities to look better, e.g., sport a tan during the winter. However, can the use of tanning beds increase vitamin D levels? The answer is "it depends." Having toured tanning salons, I found that most beds do not use UVB light. (Ultraviolet A lights are the most common bulbs but they do not stimulate vitamin D production.) If you are using a tanning facility, ask specifically for a bed that only provides UVB light.

Using indoor UVB light is an individual choice. Personally, I have not been inclined to utilize indoor tanning. I opt for limited, outdoor UVB exposure and oral vitamins D and K2 supplementation.

Food

Many Western diets are not rich in fatty fish caught in the wild. Foods that naturally contain vitamin D include salmon, mackerel, sardines, and cod liver oil. (However, cod liver oil contains a large amount of vitamin A, potentially disrupting vitamin D's processing. Please see Chapter 3.)

A number of foods are enriched with vitamin D, or cholecalciferol. Common vitamin D-fortified foods in the United States and the United Kingdom are milk, cereals, and fruit juices but they only contain small amounts of vitamin D. Enriched foods most likely will not effectively treat a vitamin D deficiency because large quantities of these foods would need to be consumed daily. For example, you would need to drink ten eight-ounce glasses of vitamin D-fortified milk daily to obtain merely 1,000 IU of vitamin D.

Vitamin D Supplementation

The most practical and effective treatment of vitamin D deficiency is to take a soft gel or liquid drop containing vitamin D3, in accordance with the Vitamin D Wellness Protocol addressed in Part IV of this book. Quality vitamin D supplements are readily available online or over-the-counter in retail stores.

The one truly effective vitamin D form is called vitamin D3 or cholecalciferol. Activated vitamin D3 is the bioidentical substance that our bodies recognize to perform essential health functions that include strengthening bones to decreasing the risk of developing cancer, heart disease, autoimmune diseases, and other serious medical conditions.

For decades, a less effective form called vitamin D2, or ergocalciferol, has been used in supplements as well as food and beverage fortification. Vitamin D2 contains synthetic compounds that are chemically altered and not well recognized by the body. Despite these facts, vitamin D2 can still be found in enriched foods and beverages as well as multi-vitamins and other supplements.

When selecting a vitamin D supplement, please read carefully the ingredient labels on vitamin supplements and fortified food and beverages to ensure you are buying D3— the only "real" vitamin D!

Beware of Prescription Vitamin D

Misperceptions about treating vitamin D deficiency still abound among medical practitioners and their patients. When treating patients for almost any medical condition, many conventional medical professionals "automatically" write prescriptions—the perceived "holy grail" for effective treatment. In turn, patients usually salute smartly by taking the prescription. However, in the case of treating vitamin D deficiency, beware of prescriptions.

At least in the United States, vitamin D deficiency is often treated with a *prescription* for "vitamin D." Guess what? The prescribed vitamin D contains the less effective form of vitamin D2 (ergocalciferol) that I addressed above. Patients are typically advised to take one prescribed 50,000 international units (IU) capsule a week, for about eight to twelve weeks. Most patients however are completely unaware that prescribed vitamin D2 comprises synthetic compounds that are chemically altered and not well recognized by the body. In my opinion taking a vitamin D *prescription* is like trying to fit a square peg into a round hole; the square peg simply does not fit! Prescribed vitamin D2 most likely will not improve your levels. Therefore, your vitamin D deficiency will not be effectively treated. You most likely will not feel better and will be wasting your time and money.

Vitamin D3 Soft Gels and Liquids Are Better Absorbed

Vitamin D is dissolved in fat. Therefore, vitamin D3 supplements in soft gel or liquid form are absorbed better than chalky tablets or chewable, fructose-laden pills. The best time to take your vitamin D3 supplement is right after your breakfast. Healthy fats, including olive oil, egg yolks, and avocado, will facilitate the absorption of vitamin D3 in your body.

Concluding Thoughts

Vitamin D supplementation is easy, effective, and inexpensive. In the next chapter you will see the other nutrients that work closely with vitamin D.

3

VITAMIN D'S PARTNERS

Vitamin D does not function alone in the body. Other vitamins and minerals interact as cofactors with activated vitamin D to perform the essential functions explained in Chapter 1. Fat-soluble vitamin K2 is dependent upon fat-soluble vitamins A and D's functions. The minerals calcium, magnesium, phosphorus, zinc, and boron also team with vitamin D.

I suggest you carefully read this chapter. The fact that specific vitamins and minerals function effectively with vitamin D does not mean that you should begin (or modify) taking supplements of these nutrients without consulting your health care practitioner. Please also consider that many of these nutrients should be obtained from your diet.

Vitamin A

The functions of vitamins A and D comprise the foundation of our health, regulating genetic activity that causes cells to make proteins required by water-soluble vitamins and minerals. Vitamin A deficiency is rare since common animal and plant foods contain this nutrient. Therefore, vitamin A supplementation is usually unnecessary.

A note of caution—when cod liver oil or retinol supplements such as retinyl acetate and retinyl palmitate are consumed on a regular basis, vitamin A toxicity may occur. Excess vitamin A in the body causes havoc because it denies vitamin D from influencing the genetic activity described above. Vitamin A supplementation may obviate the wonderful benefits of vitamin D. Please be careful!

Vitamin K2

Vitamins K2 and D partner to build and maintain strong bones and teeth as well as fight cardiovascular disease (CVD). Vitamin D's functions include regulating calcium absorption in the intestines to maintain bones and dental health. However, once calcium enters the blood stream, vitamin D relinquishes control of the mineral's destination to a less-known nutrient called vitamin K2—one of the Vitamin D Wellness Protocol trio—that moves calcium out of the arteries and into the bones and teeth.

Let's take a look at vitamin K2 and how it complements vitamin D. Like vitamins A and D, vitamin K belongs to a family of fat-soluble nutrients. Two distinct forms of vitamin K offer medical value: phylloquinone and menaquinone.

Phylloquinone or vitamin K1 is present in all green plants that acquire energy from sunlight. Green leafy vegetables including spinach, kale, collard greens, broccoli, and Brussels sprouts abound with vitamin K1. Clotting blood is primarily vitamin K1's life-saving benefit. Vitamin K1 constantly recycles in the body, so deficiency is rare.

Menaquinone or vitamin K2 differs greatly from K1. First, there are two forms of vitamin K2: menaquinone-4 (MK-4) found in *grass-fed* animal protein including meat, egg yolk, butter, some cheeses, and calf's liver. A more potent form of menaquinone, called vitamin K2 (MK-7), is abundant in a fermented soybean called natto.

Health benefits of adequate vitamin K2 levels include potential prevention of osteoporosis, arterial plaque, and dental cavities. Vitamin K2 moves calcium to the bones and teeth, as well as sweeps calcium from soft tissue lining such as the arteries. Specifically, vitamin K2 activates proteins (osteocalcin and MGP (matrix gla protein)), which are produced by vitamin D that facilitate moving calcium to where it belongs: the bones and teeth.

Low vitamin K2 levels, however, are common and may pose health risks. First, vitamin K2 receptors need regular replenishment as they are not recycled in the body. Second, the vitamin's natural sources are lacking in most diets. Owing to the reliance on industrial farming in many parts of the world, many people are low in vitamin K2 When insufficient vitamin K2 is in the blood stream, calcium can linger along arterial pathways potentially causing calcification, the process whereby calcium deposits form plaque accumulating in the cardiovascular system.

Supplementing with adequate vitamin D and K2 balances calcium metabolism. The concept of "balance" is important: one can enjoy optimal vitamin D levels but unknowingly have a vitamin K2 deficiency, a potential recipe for CVD development. Unless you ingest *grass-fed* animal products or soy-laden natto on a regular basis, consider taking a daily K2 supplement that does not contain soy products. (For example, soy can interfere with thyroid medication.) Some experts recommend a daily dose between 90 and 120 mcg. WARNING: Some anticoagulant medications (blood thinners such as warfarin) block the action of vitamin K. If you are taking any blood thinning medication, please check with your health care professional before adding *any form of vitamin K* to your body.

Calcium

The essential mineral calcium is the best known of vitamin D's partners. Vitamin D regulates calcium's absorption in the intestines so it can contribute to bone and dental health.

Calcium deficiency tends to be uncommon as most Western diets contain sufficient calcium including dairy products, leafy green vegetables, and fish products. Calcium supplementation, however, remains a topic of debate within the medical community. While calcium is essential to the bones and teeth, this mineral can linger throughout the body, potentially causing calcification in soft tissue including the kidneys and cardiovascular system.

If you are taking a calcium supplement, you may want to reconsider. Since understanding the danger of calcification of soft tissues, I have not taken a calcium supplement because my serum calcium level is within normal range. Furthermore, I consume a daily vitamin K2 supplement to increase the likelihood that the calcium in my body is moved from the bloodstream to my bones and teeth.

Magnesium

The mineral magnesium is a member of the Vitamin D Wellness Protocol trio, which includes vitamins D3 and K2. In particular, magnesium is essential to vitamin D's metabolism and absorption. An abundance of medical literature indicates that magnesium is one of the most important elements in maintaining good health. Its benefits include energy production, protection of the nervous system, improvement of muscle function, and a decrease in cardiovascular disease risk. Low magnesium levels may impair the conversion of circulating vitamin D to the activated form, denying your body vitamin D's amazing health benefits.

In today's world of fast food and pharmaceutical drugs, magnesium deficiency is common. Many diets lack natural sources of magnesium including green leafy vegetables, legumes, seeds, and nuts. Furthermore, prolific use of prescription drugs including antibiotics, proton pump inhibitors, and osteoporosis medications contribute to depletion of the body's magnesium levels. A daily magnesium supplement of at least 400 mg may boost your levels of this important mineral.

Phosphorus

Phosphorus (phosphate) is a mineral that interacts with activated vitamin D and parathyroid hormone to help maintain the balance of calcium. A wide variety of foods such as beef, chicken, eggs, seafood, legumes, nuts, grains, and dairy products contain ample amounts of phosphorus. Phosphorus imbalance is rare except for persons with excess or extremely low blood calcium or kidney disorders. Unless encouraged by a health care practitioner, phosphorus supplementation is not recommended.

Zinc

The essential mineral zinc works with activated vitamin D to bolster the immune system and influences healthy cell function. Zinc is commonly found in shellfish, red meats, beans, poultry, and nuts. Although zinc deficiency is rare, some people choose to supplement with it, about 50 mg per day.

Boron

The trace mineral boron is essential to activated vitamin D's metabolism as well as the breakdown of calcium and magnesium. Boron is contained in fruits, vegetables, seeds, nuts, and other foods produced in plants. Deficiency of boron is rare as its sources are common in most diets. Some people choose to supplement boron but for the majority of persons it is unnecessary.

Concluding Thoughts

Vitamin D functions in concert with fat-soluble vitamins A and K2 as well as a number of minerals. To reap the health benefits of vitamin D, you should be aware of its biochemical partners, specifically vitamin K2 and magnesium, which are included in Part IV's Vitamin D Wellness Protocol. The next chapter addresses how to test each vitamin D partner as well as parathyroid hormone.

4

TESTING

Testing your vitamin D level is paramount to achieving and maintaining safe optimal status. In addition, testing specific vitamin D partners or related biochemicals may be a good idea depending on your individual situation. Remember that vitamin D and its cofactors must be *balanced* in order to be effective.

Except where noted, the words "testing" and "test" means blood is collected in your medical professional's office or at home, and fasting prior to the test is not required. Reference ranges of biochemicals vary from laboratory to laboratory so please use the numbers here only as a general guide. As always, I recommend undergoing testing under the care of your health care professional.

Vitamin D

Vitamin D is the most important test to establish a vitamin D baseline and monitor any changes. The gold standard test for vitamin D is called **25(OH)D** or 25-hydroxyvitamin D where your available, or circulating, vitamin D (calcidiol) in the bloodstream is measured. The optimal range is considered 100 to 150 ng/mL (250 to 375 nmol/L) unless you have liver or kidney issues.

Another vitamin D test is called 1,25(OH)D or 1,25-dihydroxyvitamin D where your activated vitamin D (calcitriol) is measured. This test is *not* the preferred test by vitamin D experts for these reasons: a) the biological half-life of calcitriol is shorter than calcidiol and b) the test is less accurate because the 1,25(OH)D is influenced by the parathyroid hormone (PTH) as well as other hormones. Ensure the 25(OH)D, *not* the 1,25(OH)D, test is ordered.

Calcium

Calcium is absorbed in the intestines by vitamin D. A more-than-optimal vitamin D level may cause too much calcium in soft tissues and organs. So, it would be a good idea to test your serum calcium, which measures the total calcium in your blood. If **serum calcium** level is more than 10.9 mg/dL, then your parathyroid hormone should be tested.

Ionized calcium is the free, most active form of calcium. You must fast for the ionized calcium test, which should be taken if excess calcium or PTH is a suspected issue. The normal rage of ionized calcium is a level between

4.64 and 5.28 mg/dL. Low ionized calcium may indicate, *inter alia*, a vitamin D deficiency and/or low parathyroid hormone (hypoparathyroidism); abnormally high ionized calcium may suggest excess calcium and/or an overactive parathyroid gland (hyperparathyroidism).

Another method to ascertain calcium status, including the amount of calcification of the arteries, is to undergo a CT (pronounced "cat") scan for your cardiac calcium. The name of the test is "**CT coronary artery calcium (CAC)" scoring**. Valid for up to five years and unknown to the majority of the public, the CAC test is easy, fast, and non-invasive, and can be scheduled at your local radiology diagnostics center. The amount of radiation exposure is about equivalent to a mammogram, and no contrast dye is required.

The encouraging news is that the American Heart Association recommended the CAC test in its November 2018 cholesterol guidelines for determining cardiac calcium risk status and the need for statins for people aged 40 to 75 years. At the time of this writing, however, many health insurance plans do not cover the cost of this test. In my opinion, the test fee (usually less than US$200) is well worth the money. This test may save your, or a loved one's, life!

Vitamin K2

Vitamin K2 partners with vitamin D to move calcium out of the blood stream, soft tissues, and organs and into the bones. There is no generally-available test to measure directly forms of vitamin K. However, a CAC test may provide insight into the effectiveness of vitamin K2 intake in your cardiovascular system. In other words, if your CAC score, serum calcium, and/or ionized calcium are low, your consumption of vitamin K2 probably is effective. If your CAC score, serum calcium, and/or ionized calcium are high, then your parathyroid hormone should be tested.

Parathyroid Hormone

Nestled behind the thyroid gland, four tiny parathyroid glands in your neck play an important role in your body: they regulate calcium. When calcium levels are too low, the glands release **parathyroid hormone (PTH)** to restore the calcium to its normal range. Conversely, when calcium levels rise, the parathyroid glands stop releasing PTH, potentially causing a range of symptoms including kidney stones and bone pain.

Three forms of PTH are assayed in this test for which fasting is required. The reference ranges are: N-terminal: 8 to 24 pg/mL; C-terminal: 50 to 330 pg/mL; and intact molecule: 10 to 65 pg/mL. If any of your PTH forms are out-of-range, then explore further options with your doctor. For example, high PTH (hyperparathyroidism) could be directly related to a low vitamin D status.

Magnesium

The mineral magnesium plays an important role in absorption of vitamin D and calcium. The two most common magnesium tests are called serum magnesium and RBC magnesium. **Serum magnesium** is often ordered by health care professionals and evaluates the amount of magnesium in the bloodstream. The "normal" optimal range for the serum magnesium test is 1.7 to 2.2 mg/dL.

The **RBC magnesium** test however is preferred, owing to its accuracy. The majority of magnesium in the body is actually absorbed in the cells; this test measures the magnesium in the RBC or "red blood cells." According to Dr. Carolyn Dean, a renowned magnesium expert, the optimal range of the RBC magnesium test is 6.0 to 6.5 mg/dL.

Phosphorus

Absorbed in the intestines, the mineral phosphorus interacts with vitamin D, calcium, and PTH. The **serum phosphorus/phosphate** test measures the amount of inorganic phosphate in the blood (Urine testing also is available.) Phosphorus deficiencies are associated, *inter alia*, with malabsorption, excess calcium, uncontrolled diabetes, and kidney disorders. The "normal" reference range for serum phosphorus/phosphate is 2.8 to 4.5 mg/dL.

Zinc

A cofactor of vitamin D, the mineral zinc can be measured by taking a plasma (not serum) blood test called "**zinc**." (Zinc is challenging to detect in blood serum as it is distributed in trace amounts to the cells.) Zinc also can be tested using a urine test or hair analysis. Zinc deficiency affects approximately two billion people across the globe. Low zinc is associated, *inter alia*, with gut health issues, autism, and mental health challenges. The "normal" reference range for the plasma zinc test is 10.0 to 17.0 μmol/L.

Boron

Boron is a little-known element that is one of vitamin D's partners. While it is not typical to supplement with boron, some people do, and testing may be in order. A "normal" reference range is fewer than 50 μg/L.

Vitamin A

Fasting is required for the **vitamin A** test that measures retinol, the animal form of vitamin A. Deficiency in vitamin A is rare in the developed world. Nonetheless, a low level may indicate malabsorption of this vitamin D partner. On the other hand, high vitamin A may suggest, *inter alia*, consumption of excess cod liver oil, which can cause unpleasant symptoms, including liver damage, bone pain, and severe drowsiness. The reference range of vitamin A is 38 to 98 mcg/dL.

Concluding Thoughts

Nature's balance of vitamin D and its cofactors works in unison with one another. For most people, testing vitamin D—the 25(OH) D test—and serum calcium every six months is adequate to monitor your Vitamin D Wellness levels. In some cases, one out-of-range measurement can lead to more tests. With that said, it is usually unnecessary to run the gamut of the tests addressed in this chapter unless ordered by your doctor. And, as we see, much of the available testing is related to balancing calcium—a vital mineral that commands "a check and balance" to ensure optimal health!

PART II

Vitamin D: Preconception and Beyond

PART II
INTRODUCTION

One of the primary reasons I wrote the second part of *Defend Your Life II* is to convey to anyone who will listen the absolutely vital role that vitamin D plays in the beginning of life. People are often surprised to learn that vitamin D is paramount *prior to conception*. Vitamin D continues to be highly significant during pregnancy, breastfeeding, and early life. As you may know from reading the first *Defend Your Life*, vitamin D remains a constant player in health throughout our entire lives. It's that simple.

- Part II of this book first addresses fertility, in other words, the health of the biological mother, and, yes, biological father before a baby is conceived. You may be surprised to learn how important vitamin D is prior to conception.

- The second chapter in Part II examines the importance of vitamin D during pregnancy and avoiding pregnancy complications. In addition, adequate maternal vitamin D helps not only the mother but her unborn child.

- The third chapter in Part II discusses the role of vitamin D in health phases of the baby: fetal, neonatal, lactation, and early childhood.

I encourage you, regardless of your own personal family status, to read Part II. The connection between mother, father, and baby is quite remarkable.

Let's first review an intriguing 2018 case study of a breastfed, one-month-old boy in Japan. The recap of this study warrants every reader's attention:

During her pregnancy, the baby boy's mother was deficient in vitamin D and suffered a variety of complications including high blood pressure, jaundice, and morning sickness. At just over thirty-seven weeks of gestation and with underdeveloped fetal growth, the infant was delivered via a cesarean section.

- The infant was born with hypocalcaemia, or low calcium, caused by his mother's vitamin D deficiency. At two months of age, he experienced abnormal rapid breathing and was diagnosed not only with a dilated left ventricle of the heart but congestive heart failure. (Corroboration with similar studies has demonstrated the association of heart disease with a calcium deficiency, caused by a vitamin D deficiency.) The good news is that boy's cardiac function was restored with "treatment" to "nearly normal" at about six months of age.

The lesson of this study is that maternal vitamin D deficiency can cause serious medical conditions, some of which cannot be treated and resolved, in babies.

Why risk the health of an innocent baby by not taking adequate vitamin D? The risk of early life complications significantly diminishes when the carrying mother is re-plete in vitamin D.

The next chapter addresses the role of vitamin D in both male and female fertility.

5

MALE AND FEMALE FERTILITY

$\mathbf{M}$y heart breaks when I hear of couples who want to conceive so badly but cannot. I just want to shout to them from the rooftops, saying, "Take vitamin D!"

Vitamin D's Role in Reproduction

Vitamin D is intricately linked to the male and female reproductive systems. The human reproductive systems comprise billions of cells. Every cell in the female and male reproductive systems contains genetic codes as well as a receptor to receive vitamin D for processing.

Cells in the female reproductive system (including the ovaries, fallopian tubes, uterus, placenta, and decidua) are replete with vitamin D receptors. The male reproductive system cells (including the testes, sperm, prostate, and urethra) also are abundant with vitamin D receptors.

When you have ample amounts of activated vitamin D in your blood, the D binds with its receptor to regulate genes in your reproductive system. For example, activated vitamin D in females controls the genes involved in estrogen production. In males, activated vitamin D regulates the genes concerned with testosterone production. (Please note that both males and females make estrogen and testosterone hormones.)

Conversely, when the cells in the reproductive systems lack activated vitamin D, genes essential to conception are not expressed. Hence, the chances of achieving successful conception are diminished.

Both Mom and Dad Need Vitamin D for Fertility

For many couples, getting pregnant and carrying a pregnancy to term present daunting challenges. Based on anecdotal success stories, word about vitamin D's positive role in fertility is trickling into social media platforms.

More importantly, scientific research indicates that the significant prevalence of vitamin D deficiency correlates to the incidences of infertility in both women and men. Over the past several years, there has been a surge in research exploring how fertility is impacted by a dearth of vitamin D.

Female Fertility and Vitamin D

- A University of Pennsylvania School of Medicine research team demonstrated that women who were vitamin D deficient when beginning fertility treatments were forty percent less like to become pregnant. This study, dated November 6, 2017, also revealed, in particular, "a reduced likelihood of successful pregnancy and delivery if polycystic ovary syndrome (PCOS) was the underlying cause of infertility."

- Citing PCOS and endometriosis as the two most frequent causes of female infertility, a research team in Italy discussed vitamin D's role in both *in vitro* and *in vivo* studies. The researchers stated that there is increasing evidence that suggests that vitamin D has a regulatory role in PCOS. In addition, vitamin D deficiency may contribute to the pathogenesis of endometriosis. The report was published in the September 2017 issue of the journal *Reviews in Endocrine and Metabolic Disorders.*

- Another Italian research team conducted a study of 335 women who were candidates for *in vitro* fertilization (IVF). Published in an August 2014 issue of *The Journal of Clinical Endocrinology & Metabolism*, the study demonstrated that the females with vitamin D levels of greater than 30 ng/mL (75 nmol/L) enjoyed the highest probability of pregnancy. The researchers concluded that vitamin D is an emerging factor influencing female fertility and IVF outcome.

Male Fertility and Vitamin D

- Research from University College Dublin in Ireland suggests that biological fathers' vitamin D status *prior to conception* plays a significant role in determining the future height and weight of their children. The research team concluded, "Paternal vitamin D intake was positively and prospectively associated with offspring's height and weight at five years old, independent of maternal characteristics, meriting further investigation of familial dietary pathways." The research team presented its findings to a European medical conference in May 2017.

- Greek researchers examined thirty years of scientific literature on the role of vitamin D in human reproduction. The accumulated evidence suggests that vitamin D is significantly involved in the reproductive systems of both sexes. Specifically, the scientists noted that vitamin D status is associated with semen quality and sperm count, motility, and morphology. Moreover, they concluded there is a positive effect of vitamin D supplementation on fertility outcomes as well as testosterone concentrations. The literature review was published in a 2013 issue of the *International Journal of Clinical Practice*.

- An Australian fertility specialist, Anne Clark, M.D., presented findings to the 2008 Fertility Society of Australia Conference that examined the role of low vitamin D in males. More than one-third of the 794 men who underwent a vitamin D blood serum test

25(OH)D were determined to be deficient in vitamin D (as well as folate). Among the couples where the male completed supplementation treatment for nutritional deficiencies (including vitamin D), more than one-half conceived naturally or with minimal treatment.

Concluding Thoughts

Why risk the health of unborn children with a vitamin D deficiency? While vitamin D status is probably not the cause of infertility, this amazing nutrient is most likely a contributing factor to the success or failure of conception.

In concert with your health care practitioner, consider following the Vitamin D Wellness Protocol in Chapter 18 until your vitamin D level is at least 50 ng/mL (125 nmol/L) before trying to conceive a baby.

Speaking of successful conception, the next chapter examines the role of vitamin D and pregnancy.

6

THE MOTHER AND A HEALTHY PREGNANCY

When a pregnant woman is asked if she would prefer a boy or a girl, her inevitable response is similar to, "I only care that my baby is healthy." Therefore, many expectant mothers do their best to have a healthy baby by leading a wholesome lifestyle and following their doctors' orders. Nonetheless, millions of babies are born with medical conditions, many of which affect these children throughout their lives.

Researching the role of vitamin D in pregnancy for this book, I blew inches of virtual dust from a page of medical correspondence reported over seven decades ago. With keen interest I read "Vitamin-D Requirements in Pregnancy," published in a 1947 edition of the prestigious *British Medical Journal*. The author Edgar Obermer, MD asserted the necessity for English pregnant women to supplement with *robust* daily doses of vitamin D.

Perhaps Dr. Obermer was ahead of his time, or today we are behind, in understanding the power of vitamin D. I think both are true. Dr. Obermer's assertion about relatively high maternal vitamin D doses accentuates vitamin D's importance during pregnancy.

Today pregnant women typically supplement with prenatal vitamins, many of which only contain enough vitamin D to prevent rickets, a re-emerging Victorian disease that I address in Chapter 7 of this book.

Unfortunately, taking prenatal vitamins without supplementing with additional vitamin D provides expectant mothers with a false sense of health for babies and themselves. In this chapter I address vitamin D's role in pregnancy, medical literature supporting the positive effect of vitamin D on expectant moms and their babies, and vitamin D supplementation guidelines for pregnant and lactating women and their infants.

As you know from reading the chapter about fertility, the female reproductive system (includes ovaries, fallopian tubes, uterus, placenta, decidua, vagina, and breasts) comprises billions of cells that contain vitamin D receptors. When we have adequate amounts of vitamin D in the cells of the female reproductive system, the vitamin D pathway genes positively affect *in utero* fetal development. Conversely, when the female reproductive system lacks activated vitamin D, genes essential to a smooth pregnancy and sound fetal health are not expressed. Hence, the risk of developing pregnancy complications and fetal medical conditions increases.

Vitamin D and a Healthy Pregnancy

British nutrition expert Sara Patience and author of the popular book *Easy Weaning*, stated, "It's important for mums to understand that their baby will be born with the same vitamin D status as themselves, therefore, if mum is vitamin D deficient during pregnancy, baby will be, too. Women, who are pregnant, or planning to become pregnant, should ensure they are vitamin D sufficient, not only to protect their own health, but also to protect the health of their baby."

I totally agree with Ms. Patience, and cannot emphasize enough that vitamin D is vital to pregnant women's health. An adequate blood serum level in expectant moms reduces the risk of pregnancy complications including preterm birth, preeclampsia, miscarriage, and gestational diabetes mellitus.

Unfortunately, low vitamin D levels are common in pregnant women. The majority of pregnant women have blood serum vitamin D levels of less than 50 ng/mL (125 nmol/L), a measurement on the lower side of "Vitamin D Wellness" adequate. Please remember that most prenatal vitamins contain only 400 to 800 IU of vitamin D, an insufficient amount of the necessary daily intake.

- Research, published in a 2018 issue of the *International Journal of Gynecology & Obstetrics*, found a prevalence of vitamin D deficiency in southern Brazil.

- The findings of a Canadian study, published in the December 2014 issue of the journal *Current Opinion in Obstetrics and Gynecology*, accentuate the importance of vitamin D to maternal health. Lead researcher

Shu-Qin Wei, MD examined scientific evidence on the role of maternal vitamin D on pregnancy that was published between January 1, 2013 and July 1, 2014. She concluded, "Recent evidence supports [that] the low maternal vitamin D status is associated with an increased risk of adverse pregnancy outcomes. Interventional studies demonstrate that the vitamin D supplementation during pregnancy optimizes maternal and neonatal status."

Vitamin D Diminishes Pregnancy Complications Risks

Grassroots Health, a non-profit, public health organization founded by Carole Baggerly, focuses on placing vitamin D research into practice. Over the past decade Grassroots Health has teamed with medical experts at the Medical University of South Carolina (MUSC) to lead a program called "Protect Our Children NOW!" that includes decreasing the incidence of **preterm births**.

- Mrs. Baggerly and her team, including MUSC medical professionals, studied 1,064 women who received prenatal care and delivered at MUSC between September 2015 and December 2016. The researchers concluded that the women who attained a vitamin D level of at least 40 ng/mL (100 nmol/L) by the time of delivery enjoyed a 62 percent lower risk of preterm births as compared to females with levels less than 20 ng/mL (50 nmol/L). The study was published in the July 24, 2017 issue of the journal *PLOS One*.

Preeclampsia only occurs only during pregnancy and causes high blood pressure that usually sets in after 20 weeks of gestation.

- Columbian researchers performed a systematic review and analysis of the plethora of scientific evidence on the role of maternal vitamin D in the development of preeclampsia. They found that the higher the vitamin D level, the lower the probability of getting preeclampsia.

- The Brazilian study cited earlier in this chapter also concluded that vitamin D deficiency was associated with preeclampsia.

A **miscarriage** (the loss of a fetus before the 20th week of gestation) is perhaps one of the worst fears of pregnant women. Approximately 15 to 20 percent of all pregnancies in the United States end in miscarriage. Similarly, about 1 in 6 pregnancies in the United Kingdom are miscarried.

- National Institutes of Health researchers concluded that vitamin D may play a protective role in pregnancy. They studied 1,191 women who had previously suffered a miscarriage. Women who planned to conceive after a pregnancy loss and had sufficient vitamin D (greater than or equal to 30 ng/mL or 75 nmol/L) were more likely to conceive and have a live birth. The report was published in the September 2018 issue of *The Lancet Diabetes & Endocrinology* journal.

- A team of Portuguese scientists systematically reviewed studies of women who had two or more miscarriages and their vitamin D status. The studies reported a high prevalence of vitamin D deficiency in women with recurrent miscarriages. The findings were published in the July 27, 2018 edition of the *American Journal of Reproductive Immunology.*

Gestational diabetes mellitus (GDM) develops in about seven percent of pregnant women. GDM may occur during a significant spike in blood sugar between the 24th and 28th weeks. If GDM is untreated, the children are at a higher risk of being overweight and developing Type 2 diabetes mellitus later in life.

- Researchers studied Australian and New Zealand pregnant women to understand better the relationship between vitamin D status and GDM. They concluded that pregnant women with a vitamin D level of greater than 32 ng/mL (81 nmol/L) at the 15th week of gestation enjoyed a decreased risk of developing GDM. The study was published on June 20, 2018 in *BMC Pregnancy & Childbirth.*

- A 2018 study examined the link between the incidences of GDM in 515 pregnant Saudi women. The research revealed a significantly higher risk of GDM among pregnant women who are deficient (less than 20 ng/mL or 50 nmol/L) in vitamin D. Results of the study were published in the April 10, 2018 issue of *BMC Pregnancy & Childbirth.*

No pregnant women look forward to the intensity of labor pain. The benefits of maternal vitamin D have been extended to decreased **labor pain.**

- On October 14, 2014, Andrew W. Geller, MD, a physician anesthesiologist at Cedars-Sinai Medical Center in Los Angeles, presented a study of vitamin D's effect on labor pain to the annual meeting of the American Society of Anesthesiologists. Dr. Geller and his team measured the vitamin D level of 93 pregnant women prior to delivery. All of the patients requested an epidural for labor pain. The researchers then measured the doses of pain medication required by each woman during labor. The quantity of pain medicine consumed by women with higher vitamin D levels was compared to those women with lower vitamin D status. The patients with lower vitamin D levels used more pain drugs than those women who enjoyed a higher vitamin D status. Dr. Geller concluded that "prevention and treatment of low vitamin D levels in pregnant women may have a significant impact on decreasing labor pain in millions of women every year."

Vitamin D Supplementation Guidelines for Pregnant Women

Remember Dr. Obermer from the beginning of this chapter? Well, over seventy years ago, he offered a surprising recommendation. Remarking that the subject of vitamin D supplementation during pregnancy "is a difficult and complex one," Dr. Obermer concludes, "In a climate like that of England every pregnant woman should be given a supplement of vitamin D doses of not less than 10,000 i.u. per day in the first seven months, and 20,000 i.u. during the 8th and 9th months."

Yet more than seven decades later, vitamin D requirements for pregnant women continue to be a topic of debate. But Dr. Obermer's words are music to my ears. It is refreshing to note that the Vitamin D Council and the Endocrine Society—both highly respected organizations—recommend upper limit vitamin D doses that almost mirror those of Dr. Obermer's.

Daily vitamin D recommendations for pregnant women are as follows:

- Vitamin D Council: 4,000-6,000 IU (Upper limit: 10,000 IU).
- Endocrine Society: 1,500-2,000 IU (Upper limit: 10,000 IU).
- Institute of Medicine (IOM): 600 IU (Upper limit: 4,000 IU).

("Upper limit" denotes the dose is safe and tolerable.)

NOTE: The IOM Food and Nutrition Board's controversial low recommendations, announced almost a decade ago, were largely based on nutritional requirements for bone health. Most vitamin D experts agree that the IOM guidelines are woefully low with regard to vitamin D. I note that the recommended daily intake of vitamin D's primary partners, magnesium and vitamin K2, were not addressed by the IOM.

Concluding Thoughts

To assert that adequate vitamin D is vital to a pregnant woman's health is to state the obvious. Pregnancy imposes exceptional demands on vitamin D availability. Both mother and child need lots of vitamin D to minimize pregnancy complications as well as maximize fetal health. In the next chapter we discuss vitamin D's connection to fetal, neonatal, lactation, and early childhood development.

7

THE BABY

Adequate vitamin D is essential to moms *and* their unborn children. So many mothers are low in D, threatening not only their health but their babies'. In this chapter we look at research about vitamin D and fetal, neonatal, and early childhood health. In addition, we will look at the role vitamin D plays in breastfeeding, or lactation.

Fetal Health

Vitamin D is vital to fetal bone and cell development.

- Dutch health scientist Dr. Marieke Weernink and her research team explored the effect of vitamin D supplementation during pregnancy and early infancy on skull formations. The scientists recommended that women in their last trimester and early infants take a daily vitamin D dose of 400 IU (an extremely low dose). The researchers discovered that pregnant mums and their infants who did not adhere to their vitamin D recommendation are linked to an increased risk of skull deformities in babies at two to four months of age. This study was published in the January 2015 issue of the journal *Maternal & Child Nutrition*.

Furthermore, medical research suggests some "seeds" of disease are sown *prior to birth*. Babies born to women with a vitamin D deficiency are more likely to develop a number of serious medical conditions including asthma, autism, cardiovascular malformation, and type 1 diabetes mellitus.

Groundbreaking research from the University of Southampton in the United Kingdom indicates that children at four years of age are likely to develop stronger muscles when their mothers enjoyed a higher maternal vitamin D during pregnancy.

- Led by Nicholas Harvey, PhD, the researchers measured the vitamin D levels of 678 mothers from the Southampton Women's Survey in the later stages of pregnancy. Four years after the babies were born, the research team measured the young children's hand-grip strength and muscle mass. The researchers found that the higher the levels of vitamin D in the mother, the higher the grip strength of her child.

The Southampton's study, published in the January 2014 issue of the *Journal of Clinical Endocrinology and*

Metabolism, suggests more far-reaching health benefits. Dr. Harvey commented,

- "These associations between maternal vitamin D and offspring muscle strength may well have consequences for later health; muscle strength peaks in young adulthood before declining in older age and low grip strength in adulthood has been associated with poor health outcomes including diabetes, falls, and fractures. It is likely that the greater muscle strength observed at four years of age in children born to mothers with higher vitamin D levels will track into adulthood, and so potentially help to reduce the burden of illness associated with loss of muscle mass in old age."

Lactation

Nature intended for newborns to obtain their nutrients, including vitamin D, from their mothers' breast milk. Breastfeeding typically provides babies with the vitamins and minerals required for healthy development. It is imperative that lactating mums *supplement daily* with adequate vitamin D.

- Medical University of South Carolina researchers, including Bruce Hollis, PhD, and Carol Wagner, MD, conducted a landmark randomized controlled trial of vitamin D supplementation during lactation. Having defined vitamin D *deficiency* as less than or equal to 20 ng/mL (50 nmol/L), the research team compared the effectiveness of maternal vitamin D supplementation with 6,400 IU daily with as low as 400 IU. The study's authors concluded that daily maternal vitamin D supplementation of 6,400 IU safely supplies adequate vitamin D in breastmilk for the nursing infant. The details of this pioneering study were published in the October 2015 issue of the journal *Pediatrics.*

Vitamin D Supplementation for Babies

According to the Vitamin D Council, if you are lactating and taking 6,000 IU of vitamin D per day, your breast milk should have enough vitamin D for your baby. If you, the mother, are taking less than 6,000 IU daily, you should give your baby vitamin D drops once a day.

Daily vitamin D supplementation guidelines for *babies* include:

- Vitamin D Council: 1,000 IU (Upper limit: 2,000 IU).
- Endocrine Society: 400-1,000 IU (Upper limit: 2,000 IU).
- Institute of Medicine: 400 IU (Upper limit: 1,000–1,500 IU).

Neonatal Health

Unfortunately, complications can occur with infants who are twenty-eight days or fewer in age. Neonatal complications may include low birth weight, sepsis, and respiratory tract infections. Once again, the positive effect of vitamin D plays a role in neonatal health.

- A Chinese research team investigated the vitamin D status of 150 neonatal patients with sepsis. The researchers found that inflammation associated with sepsis was significantly decreased after one vitamin D treatment (a 10,000-IU injection) over a seventy-two hour period! The study was published in the August 2018 edition of the journal *Experimental and Therapeutic Medicine.*

- An earlier Chinese study, published in a 2016 issue of the *Chinese Journal of Contemporary Pediatrics,* concluded that neonatal vitamin D is directly connected to maternal vitamin D.

Early Childhood Health: Rickets

I cannot overemphasize the importance of adequate vitamin D to early life health.

For starters, let's look at the disease called rickets, briefly addressed in Chapter 1. Triggered by vitamin D deficiency, rickets usually begins to affect babies from three to eighteen months of age. Symptoms include skeletal deformities, curvature of the spine, and generalized muscle weakness and lethargy.

Rickets causes bone deformity, a condition that was referenced in records as far back as 900 BC. Fast forward several centuries to the mid-1600s when scientific reporting of rickets began, owing to the disease's rampancy in England and other parts of Europe. The prevalence of rickets peaked during the Industrial Revolution in the United States and northern Europe when so many people transitioned from working in the fields to indoor factories.

The debilitating disease all but disappeared in the twentieth century, thanks to the routine administration of cod liver oil, an excellent anti-rachitic agent. But, shockingly, rickets has reemerged in the twenty-first century, owing to, *inter alia*, lack of sunlight exposure, liberal use of sunscreen, as well as inadequate vitamin D in lactation milk.

Today researchers still explore how to manage rickets.

- Published in a January 2018 issue of the journal *Bone Reports*, a study performed by South African researchers concluded that a deficiency of calcium also plays a part in the development of rickets.

In addition to nutritional calcium, babies and young children also need dietary phosphorus, protein-rich animal and plant foods, in order to build strong bones.

Concluding Thoughts

Reflecting on Dr. Harvey's wise words near the beginning of this chapter, vitamin D in pregnancy and early in life "will track into adulthood." They form an appropriate segues into Part III where we discuss vitamin D's amazing potential role in preventing and treating a variety of medical conditions.

ABCs of Vitamin D Health

PART III
INTRODUCTION

The third part of *Defend Your Life II* addresses vitamin D's protective and treatment roles for a variety of serious medical conditions that I address as the ABC's of Vitamin D discovery/research. The subjects are: Alzheimer's, asthma, autism, autoimmune diseases, bone diseases, cancer, and cardiovascular disease.

Part III is based on the most recent *human* research available at the time of this writing. I emphasize "human" because vitamin D-related studies and trials about *us* are much more credible than animal research. I note however that research conducted on animals is an important step in the assessment of vitamin D's efficacy but should not be the basis of supplementing with the vitamin.

In 2014, I attended the annual Vitamin D Workshop ironically assembled in the bowels of a dark conference center tucked beneath the banks of the Chicago River. More than 250 people from around the world convened in rainy Chicago to share and discuss the latest laboratory research on vitamin D. I had the pleasure of meeting "vitamin D people" from several continents who shared my passion about the potential health powers of vitamin D. My participation provided insight into the minute detail of the biochemistry involved to ascertain vitamin D's mechanisms of action that I addressed in Chapter 1.

As you peruse this part of *Defend Your Life II*, you will see how human research suggests that enjoying an adequate vitamin D level may indeed decrease the risk of developing some life-threatening diseases. Furthermore, scientific studies indicate that vitamin D, at least in some cases, may have the capability to treat disease. Enjoy!

8

ALZHEIMER'S DISEASE

The number of Alzheimer's patients is growing at an alarming rate. Nearly 50 million people worldwide have developed Alzheimer's Disease (AD), according to the organization Alzheimer's Disease International. Moreover, incidences of the deadly disease are expected to increase significantly over the next few decades.

About 5,700,000 Americans are living with AD today, according to the Alzheimer's Association. Furthermore, between the years 2000 and 2015, deaths from AD have increased a whopping 123 percent! Regrettably, by the year 2050, the number of Americans suffering from AD is projected to increase almost three-fold.

The medical community's views about why the prevalence of AD is rising at a staggering rate remain varied. Many believe genetics and environmental pollutants may serve as risk factors. Some believe the predominance of vitamin D deficiency may be linked to the mounting incidences of AD. In fact, scientific research indicates that the majority of Alzheimer patients have low levels of vitamin D.

But first, let's understand what happens to the brain when Alzheimer's strikes it.

The Brain on Alzheimer's

The sheer complexity of the human brain is daunting. A healthy adult brain contains approximately 100 billion nerve cells, called neurons, which connect at more than 100 *trillion* points in the central nervous system.

The adverse effects of Alzheimer's on the brain are obvious to medical personnel interpreting the images. First, the brain of an AD patient is smaller than one of a healthy adult. The decreased brain size is a result of the brain tissue containing significantly fewer neurons. Second, abnormal clusters of amyloid-beta protein fragments, called plaques, collect between nerve cells in the brain. Third, dead or dying neurons, called tangles, are visibly present in the brain of an AD patient.

Signals traveling through the brain's extensive neural network form the basis of memories, thoughts, and feelings. When plaques and tangles develop in the brain, the signaling essential to cognitive function becomes disrupted. Consequently, brain cells are destroyed, resulting in progressive cognitive issues including memory loss, poor decision-making and behavioral problems.

One in three Americans over the age of 65 with AD or another dementia will die. Dementia kills more than breast and prostate cancers combined!

Vitamin D's Beneficial Effects on the Brain

Vitamin D crosses the blood-brain barrier. And every one of the 100 billion or so neurons in the brain includes a vitamin D receptor (VDR) that influences cognitive health. In order to regulate specific brain functions, the VDR in these cells must be turned on by receiving activated vitamin D. Without sufficient vitamin D to activate its receptors, the neurons cannot work properly.

Activated vitamin D affects the development of neurons as well as their maintenance and survival, by regulating the synthesis of nerve growth factor.

Remember those plaques and tangles that disrupt the brain's intricate signaling system? Neuro-protective effects of vitamin D also include the modulation of signal stability within the brain's complex neural network.

The Association of Vitamin D Deficiency and Alzheimer's

An abundance of research connects vitamin D deficiency, a condition that is highly prevalent in adults aged 65 years and above, to cognitive decline. So I explored the research of vitamin D's role with regard to the **risk** of AD development to understand more about the association.

- A Polish study, published in the August 18, 2018 issue of the journal *Nutrients*, investigated whether vitamin D is associated with the cognitive function of geriatric patients. The researchers found that "higher vitamin D levels" are "independently associated with better

cognitive performance and lower risk of dementia."
They recommended that vitamin D deficiency in geriatric patients should gain more medical attention, or
become a marker, when diagnosing "cognitive dysfunction and dementia."

- Dutch researchers explored vitamin D and risk of
  dementia within the decades-long, population-based
  Rotterdam Study. Studying thousands of participants,
  the research team found that lower vitamin D levels
  were associated with a higher risk of dementia. The
  research was published in a 2017 issue of the *Journal of
  Alzheimer's Disease*.

- International experts gathered at an invitational sum-
  mit on "Vitamin D and Cognition in Older Adults"
  to provide "clear" guidance to researchers and clini-
  cians about the role of vitamin D in Alzheimer's. They
  agreed that vitamin D deficiency (a blood serum level
  < 30ng/mL or 75 nmol/L) increases the risk of cognitive decline and dementia in adults aged 65 and older.
  Their report was published in the January 2015 edition
  of the prestigious *Journal of Internal Medicine*.

Could Vitamin D Prevent Alzheimer's?

We do not know for certain that vitamin D can prevent
Alzheimer's or dementia. However, research suggests that
Alzheimer's begins its development many years before AD
symptoms are apparent.

- An Australian team of researchers explored the vitamin D status of patients from the Women's Healthy Ageing Project over a decade. Specifically, the team assessed midlife vitamin D and cognition ten years later. The researchers concluded that even a small amount of vitamin D (greater than 10 ng/mL or 25 nmol/L) "is associated with improved aspects of executive function in ageing [sic]." Their findings, reported in the January 2018 issue of the scientific journal *Maturitas*, also highlighted that taking vitamin D at midlife "could be neuroprotective against cognitive decline."

- A French-led research team studied 916 participants aged 65 or older, who did not initially present with dementia or AD, over a period up to twelve years. The report, published in a 2017 issue of the journal *Alzheimers & Dementia*, suggested that "maintaining adequate vitamin D status in older age could contribute to slow down cognitive decline and to delay or prevent the onset of dementia."

- A breakthrough study, published the September 8, 2015 edition of the journal *Neurology*, revealed that Alzheimer's may develop 18 years before clinical diagnosis. These findings suggest that we may be able to prevent this deadly disease. They also indirectly hint at the need for humans to be vitamin D-rich throughout life.

Concluding Thoughts

The escalating rates of Alzheimer's suggest that your life—in some fashion—will most likely be negatively impacted by this deadly disease. Considering the association between vitamin D deficiency and Alzheimer's, I encourage readers of all ages to consider seriously adequate daily supplementation with vitamin D and its partners, magnesium and vitamin K2. In other words, please consider following the Vitamin D Wellness Protocol stated in Chapter 18 to decrease your risk of developing this deadly disease.

Please note that "dementia" encompasses a spectrum of brain-related symptoms that adversely affect memory and thinking. AD is a specific form, or subset, of dementia that spans impaired thought, impeded speech, and confusion.

9

ASTHMA

The association between asthma and vitamin D has recently garnered supportive attention in the research world. First, let's look briefly at the condition:

More than 235 million people worldwide—children and adults—suffer from asthma, a potentially lethal disease. In 2015, about 383,000 persons died from asthma, according to the World Health Organization (WHO).

Asthma is a chronic, non-communicable disease that inhibits the lungs from moving air in and out of them. When bronchial airways in the lungs become *inflamed* and swollen, these tubes narrow, decreasing the air flow.

The global medical and scientific communities do not completely understand the cause of asthma. The most likely risk factors encompass environmental exposure to particles or substances that may provoke allergic reactions or irritate the pulmonary airways.

What is the Link between Vitamin D and Asthma?

While the exact cause of asthma remains unknown, the mechanisms of action between asthma and vitamin D have been explored. Inflammation is a reaction from asthma. We know that vitamin D reduces inflammation. Furthermore, we recognize that vitamin D helps to produce T-cells that fight invader cells. In other words, a healthy immune system may reduce inflammation as well as decrease the risk of acquiring an infection such as influenza and the common cold.

A Canadian study of nearly 4,000 individuals aged 13 to 69 years revealed that those with a vitamin D level of less than 20 ng/mL (50 nmol/L) were more likely to have asthma than those subjects who had a greater level. This research was published in the September 2015 issue of the *Journal of Asthma.*

Can Adequate Vitamin D Prevent Asthma?

We know from previous chapters in this book how adequate vitamin D supplementation may decrease the risk of developing illnesses during childhood.

Published in the June 2018 edition of *Clinical and Translational Medicine*, a study, conducted by Vanderbilt University researchers, indicates that a "sufficient prenatal vitamin D level" is a common and modifiable risk factor for childhood development of asthma.

A research team from the University of Aberdeen in Scotland discovered that supplementing with vitamin D during pregnancy decreased the risk of developing asthma at the age of 10. Their findings were reported in the April 2015 issue of the *European Respiratory Journal.*

Can Adequate Vitamin D Treat Asthma?

Recent published research exudes evidence about the positive role of vitamin D supplementation in treating asthma in both children and adults.

- A clinical trial of vitamin D and asthma, published in the September 2017 edition of the journal *Chest*, revealed that vitamin D reduced asthma attacks by 300 percent in children!

- Researchers at Cairo University in Egypt measured the vitamin D level of 115 adults, 82 of whom had asthma. By administering an active form of vitamin D called alfacalcidol, the scientists found not only improved lung function but significantly reduced asthma severity. They also noted that vitamin D deficiency was more common in asthma patients. The results of this randomized clinical trial were published in the May 2017 issue of the *Annals of Allergy, Asthma & Immunology.*

- A team of Italian scientists evaluated a year-long benefit of vitamin D supplementation for 119 asthmatic adults. The results, reported in the November 2017 edition of the journal *Nutrients*, indicated a reduction in asthma "exacerbations."

- An international team of researchers conducted a systematic review of studies pertaining to vitamin D supplementation's effect on acute respiratory tract infections. As these types of infection can ignite asthma attacks, vitamin D supplementation can diminish the risk of developing a cold or influenza, thus reducing asthmatic symptoms. This research was published in the prestigious *British Journal of Medicine* in February 2017.

Concluding Thoughts

Asthma is a serious medical condition that can severely affect quality of life and cause death. About ten Americans die each day from asthma.

When I wrote this chapter, I had a dear friend in mind. For the majority of her life, she has suffered from asthma. My hope is that she continues to follow the Vitamin D Wellness Protocol and finds relief from her symptoms.

Credible medical research positively links asthma with vitamin D. As you see from the recent research cited in this chapter, it behooves asthmatics to consider adequate supplementation of vitamin D and its partners as described in Chapter 18.

10

AUTISM

An alarming number of children—in the United States and other industrialized countries—are being diagnosed with Autism Spectrum Disorder (ASD) or autism, a group of complex brain disorders. In 2018, experts estimated that 1 in 59 children are identified with ASD, according to the Centers for Disease Control and Prevention. This statistic represents a 15 percent increase in prevalence over the previous two years.

The medical and scientific communities' views about the cause of the escalating rate of ASD remain varied. Many believe genetics and environmental pollutants may serve as risk factors. Others conjecture that the identification of the disorder has become more accurate Some think that vitamin D deficiency may be linked to the mounting cases of autism.

Vitamin D and Brain Development

The connection between brain development and vitamin D is well known to vitamin D experts. Every cell in the brain includes a vitamin D receptor (VDR) that controls genes that influence brain development. To regulate gene expression, the VDR in the brain cells must be turned on by receiving activated vitamin D. Without adequate vitamin D to activate its receptors, the brain cannot function properly.

For example, a landmark study, published in the June 2014 edition of the *FASEB Journal*, California presented evidence that activated vitamin D regulates the production of the neurotransmitter serotonin. (Serotonin acts as a growth factor during early brain development.) The researchers noted that low concentrations of serotonin are found in central brain blood levels of ASD patients but are higher in the peripheral blood levels (in other words, outside the blood-brain barrier). Moreover, the scientists stated that vitamin D supplementation "is a practical and affordable solution to help prevent autism and possibly ameliorate some symptoms of the disorder."

The Association of Vitamin D with Autism

Reported in the March 2018 issue of the *Journal of Bone and Mineral Research*, a Chinese study compared the vitamin D levels of 310 ASD children with 1,240 typically developing children. The average vitamin D level "was significantly lower in children with ASD compared to controls." This same Chinese research team also examined the association between neonatal vitamin D status and the risk of developing ASD. The researchers concluded, "Neonatal vitamin D status was significantly associated with the risk of ASD and intellectual disability."

Vitamin D: Treatment for Autism

An international scientific team explored the effect of vitamin D supplementation on three children with ASD. The researchers found that ASD core symptoms responded well to the supplementation. When vitamin D administration stopped, the ASD symptoms reappeared. The study's results demonstrated—albeit with an extremely small sample—that primary ASD symptoms fluctuated in severity with changes in the children's vitamin D levels. Published in the April 8, 2018 issue of the journal *Nutritional Neuroscience*, the study indicated that vitamin D blood levels of up to 100 ng/mL may be optimal for treating ASD patients.

A more remarkable study, reported in the October 2016 issue of the journal *Nutritional Neuroscience*, examined 122 Egyptian children (aged 3 to 9) with ASD. Eighty-three children completed three months of daily vitamin D treatment (ranging between 300 IU and 5,000 IU). Eighty percent of these children had a "significantly improved outcome": primarily in CARS (Childhood Autism Rating Scale) scores and "aberrant behavior checklists…that measure behavior, stereotypy persistent repetitive behavior], eye contact, and attention span." The researchers concluded, "Vitamin D is inexpensive, readily available and safe. It may have beneficial effects in ASD subjects, especially when the final serum level is more than 40 ng/mL."

The association between vitamin D levels and treatment of autism is real, folks. A quick scan of autism assessment scores such as CARS with and without vitamin D supplementation is indeed eyebrow-raising.

I highly encourage parents of autistic children to consider nutritional supplementation that includes daily vitamin D3, vitamin K2, and magnesium: yes, the three nutrients in the Vitamin D Wellness Protocol in Chapter 18.

Let's take this a step further: Several years ago John J. Cannell, MD, founder of the non-profit renowned organization called the Vitamin D Council, wrote a superb book entitled *Autism Causes: Prevention and Treatment* that included his daily nutritional recommendations for treating autism. They include 5,000 to 15,000 IU of vitamin D3, 125 to 500 mg of magnesium, 80 mcg of vitamin K2, and 12 mg of zinc. (Please see "Additional Resources" for further information on Dr. Cannell's autism book.)

In 2015, I was invited to speak about vitamin D at the Autism One conference in Chicago. Greatly honored to present vitamin D research to parents of autistic children, I talked about the new—at the time—research on how vitamin D supplementation reduced the severity of ASD symptoms.

One of the studies that I presented looked at three major autism assessments with regard to scores pre- and post-vitamin D supplementation: Autism Behavior Checklist, CARS, and Clinical Global Severity of Illness scale. The questionnaire scores before and after vitamin D supplementation demonstrated obvious improvement. This *Pediatrics* study was published in January 2015.

Concluding Thoughts

Can vitamin D reduce the risk of developing autism? I do think low vitamin D levels in pregnant moms may contribute to the development of the disorder. Taking one step further, if two people intend to have a baby, they should try to have optimal levels of vitamin D prior to conception.

In the next chapter we explore vitamin D's role regarding autoimmune diseases including lupus and multiple sclerosis.

11

AUTOIMMUNE DISEASES

An autoimmune disease happens when one's immune system attacks itself. These diseases are becoming more prevalent these days

An estimated 50 million Americans suffer from an autoimmune disease, according to the American Autoimmune Related Diseases Association, Inc. And this number is increasing not only in the United States but worldwide. Why the surge?

The answer, in part at least, takes me back to 2007 when I was attending my first medical seminar to learn how to improve my health. (This information contributed to improving health as well as inspiring my first book entitled *Defend Your Life*.)

To this day, I get goosebumps recalling a map of the world was displayed for the seminar participants including mostly medical doctors. The map indicated that multiple sclerosis was prevalent *only outside the equatorial region.* People who lived in areas near the sunny equator rarely develop MS!

Moreover, the use of sunscreen products has risen, denying us vitamin D.

This was my first "aha" moment during my medical journey. The coincidence between the lack of MS and an abundance of sun light—the natural source of vitamin D— was uncanny. Since that time, I have researched the medical literature about vitamin D and MS, as well as other autoimmune diseases. The results are enlightening.

Having explained the role of vitamin D and sunlight in Chapter 2, I discuss vitamin D's association with several common autoimmune diseases: Type 1 diabetes mellitus, Hashimoto's thyroiditis, lupus (or SLE), multiple sclerosis (MS), and rheumatoid arthritis (RA).

What is Autoimmunity?

There are two types of immune systems in the human body: innate and adaptive. We are born with an innate immune system to protect against general attackers that could cause disease. After birth we begin to develop an adaptive immune system. This system comprises the body's intricate network of antibodies (B-cells) and special types of white blood cells (called sensitized lymphocytes or T-cells) to thwart new as well as previous invaders, including viruses, bacteria, and medication. When the adaptive immune system is not strong enough to fight external threats such as infections, it can go awry by signaling antibodies and T-cells to attack healthy cells. This response is called *autoimmunity*—when the body's immune cells attack its own healthy cells.

Vitamin D Helps Regulate the Adaptive Immune System

Scientific research over the past three decades solidifies the connection between vitamin D and autoimmunity. Vitamin D plays an integral role in the regulation of the adaptive immune system. Adequate vitamin D in our bodies can protect us from autoimmunity because adaptive immune cells contain vitamin D receptors (VDR). These receptors are attached to the surface of the adaptive immune system's antibodies and sensitized lymphocytes.

The VDR act as "gate keepers" by signaling what external substances, e.g., components of medications, can enter a healthy cell. However, the VDR must be replete with vitamin D to effectively regulate adaptive immunity. When the VDR receive adequate amounts of vitamin D, they enable the adaptive immune system to function properly by attacking new and previous invaders.

When the VDR attached to the adaptive immune system's cells do not contain sufficient activated vitamin D to attack invaders, autoimmunity may kick in, causing the death of healthy immune cells. Thus, low vitamin D levels may lead to the development of autoimmune diseases including Type 1 diabetes mellitus, Hashimoto's thyroiditis, lupus, MS, and RA.

Type 1 Diabetes Mellitus

Type 1 diabetes mellitus—affecting about 1.25 million Americans with increasing prevalence worldwide—is a chronic autoimmune disease where the pancreas is unable to make insulin in its beta islet cells. The body's immune system attacks and destroys the pancreatic beta islet cells until insulin can no longer be produced. Insulin, a vital hormone, regulates blood sugar (glucose) levels in muscle and other tissue cells to help control energy. The lack of insulin creates elevated blood sugar.

Type 1 diabetes usually occurs during childhood or adolescence but can strike at any age. Once type 1 diabetes has developed, it never goes away. Type 1 diabetes' onset translates to a *forever* regimen: measuring blood sugar at least four times a day, injecting or pumping insulin as needed, monitoring carbohydrate intake, and exercising.

Vitamin D has the potential to prevent type 1 diabetes. The pancreatic beta islet cells, that make insulin, contain VDR that receive and produce *activated* vitamin D (calcitriol). So what does this mean? Activated vitamin D protects the beta islet cells by reducing the production of cytokines, substances that destroy beta islet cells, and may prevent the development of type 1 diabetes mellitus.

A landmark study, published in a 2018 issue of the journal *Diabetes*, found that children with low vitamin D levels were more likely to develop type 1 diabetes mellitus. Led by Dr. Jill Norris of the University of Colorado, the international research team followed 8,676 children in the United States and Europe. These children had a previously identified genetic risk for developing type 1 diabetes mellitus. The researchers took circulating vitamin D samples from each child every three-to-six months from infancy, up to four years. Ultimately, a total of 376 children developed an autoimmunity to beta islet cells which causes type 1 diabetes mellitus. *The lesson learned is that infants and children who enjoy adequate vitamin D levels may see a reduction in risk to develop a disease that affects them daily for life.*

Hashimoto's Thyroiditis

Discovered over one hundred years ago by a Japanese physician, Hashimoto's thyroiditis is an autoimmune disease that attacks and damages the thyroid gland causing low thyroid activity or hypothyroidism.

Hashimoto's (or "Hashi's" for short) is the most common thyroid disorder in the world. About one to two percent of Americans suffer from Hashimoto's thyroiditis. The disease is four times more common in women than men.

The thyroid, a butterfly-shaped gland located in your neck, regulates your metabolism and affects every cell in your body. When your thyroid is not working properly, your hormones can become unbalanced, potentially causing symptoms including weight gain or loss and chronic fatigue as well as autoimmune disease and cancer.

Vitamin D receptors (VDR) are present in the cells of the pituitary, the pea-sized gland located at the base of the brain that controls your thyroid. The pituitary produces a hormone called thyroid stimulating hormone (TSH) that signals your thyroid gland to make thyroid hormones (T3 and T4). Thyroid hormone constantly circulates throughout your body, regulating metabolism. Inadequate or excessive thyroid hormone can wreak havoc to your health, culminating in hypothyroidism.

Unsurprisingly, scientific research indicates that low vitamin D levels are common in Hashi's patients. For example, a 2017 case-control study published in the *Egyptian Journal of Immunology* found that vitamin D was deficient in 76.6 percent of Hashimoto's thyroiditis patients.

Understanding the regulating effects of VDR in our cells, I surmise that the amount of activated vitamin D in the pituitary's VDR may be connected to the release of thyroid hormones. However, further investigation needs to be conducted to say whether vitamin D supplementation can prevent or treat Hashimoto's.

Lupus (SLE)

Lupus ("systemic lupus erythematosus" or SLE) is a chronic autoimmune disease that attacks the body's healthy cells, tissues, and organs. This disease results in severe inflammation, fatigue, and, in some cases, death.

About 1.5 million Americans and over five million persons globally, suffer from a form of lupus, according to the Lupus Foundation of America. Ninety percent of persons diagnosed with lupus are women, many of whom are in their reproductive years.

Research suggests that adequate vitamin D in the body may protect against the development of SLE. Genetic and environmental factors as well as vitamin D deficiency have been linked to lupus. Sensitivity to sunlight, the primary source of vitamin D, is common among SLE patients.

Scientific research indicates a high prevalence of

vitamin D deficiency among those persons suffering lupus. For example, a Singaporean research team found that vitamin D deficiency is highly prevalent in SLE patients. Furthermore, the study, published in the August 10, 2018 edition of the *International Journal of Molecular Sciences*, also revealed that circulating vitamin D levels may be correlated with increased disease activity of SLE including fatigue, cardiovascular risk, and cognitive impairment.

Multiple Sclerosis (MS)

Multiple sclerosis (MS) befits a disease of modern civilization, one of sun avoidance. Initially identified by French neurologist Jean-Martin Charcot in 1868, MS is a chronic, neurological autoimmune disorder that damages the myelin sheath, the multiple layers of fatty tissue that surround and protect the nerves in the brain, spinal cord, and optic nerves. When the myelin sheath is intact, electrical impulses are carried through the nerves with accuracy and speed. When the myelin sheath is damaged (sclerosis is the scar tissue formed by damaged myelin), the nerves do not conduct electrical impulses normally. The impulses are distorted or interrupted, resulting in a range of symptoms including numbness, blindness, paralysis, and brain damage. MS also can result in death.

Despite the identification of MS one-hundred-fifty years ago, MS has no cure. Over 2.3 million people around the world have been diagnosed with MS including about one million Americans. Women are to two to three times more likely to develop MS than men. Although MS is usually diagnosed between the ages of 20 and 50, the disease can strike at any age. In addition, Caucasian women of northern European descent are more frequently diagnosed with MS than African Americans, Hispanics, and Asians.

To this day I always think of my cousin Judith Ann when I hear the words "multiple sclerosis." If you've read the MS chapter in the original *Defend Your Life,* you know my cousin's heartfelt story. But there is some encouraging news. Since I penned *Defend Your Life* an enormous amount of research on the association between MS and vitamin D has emerged.

Can we prevent MS before it develops? A Danish-led research team investigated the direct association between neonatal vitamin D levels and the risk of developing MS. Published in a January 2017 issue of the journal *Neurology,* the study concluded that "low concentrations of neonatal vitamin D are associated with an increased risk of MS." The publication of this study prompted a comment in a subsequent issue of *Neurology* , "A gestational dose of vitamin D per day keeps the MS doctor away."

As part of the Environmental Risk Factors in MS Study, researchers at the University of Bergen in Norway sought to understand better the association between MS and sun exposure measures by studying a total of 1,660 MS patients and 3,050 subjects from Norway and Italy. The researchers' findings included significant connections between infrequent summer outdoor activity and sunscreen use and an increased risk of MS. Published in the January 10, 2014 issue of *Multiple Sclerosis,* the study's conclusion stated, "Converging evidence from different measures underlines the beneficial effect of sun exposure on MS risk."

The scientific community is delivering hope to MS

patients by investigating vitamin D intake as a *treatment* for the disease. Research suggests that higher vitamin D levels are associated with reduced disease activity in MS sufferers.

Australian researchers analyzed twelve studies that involved 950 patients to understand better the therapeutic role of vitamin D in multiple sclerosis. The research team concluded that vitamin D supplementation may have a role in treating MS. The study was published in a December 2018 issue of the *Journal of Neurology*.

Dr. Alberto Ascherio (I had the pleasure of meeting Dr. Ascherio at a 2014 vitamin D research workshop) of Harvard University's School of Public Health and colleagues concluded that vitamin D appears to be connected with MS disease activity and progression in patients who experienced an initial episode suggestive of MS and were treated with interferon β-1b. The researchers found that 20 ng/mL-increases of vitamin D levels within the first 12 months of experiencing an initial episode predicted a 57 percent lower rate of new active lesions as well as a lower risk of relapse. In addition, the results included a 25 percent decrease in annual T2 lesion volume and a 0.41 percent lower yearly loss in brain volume over four years. The Harvard study was electronically published on January 20, 2014 in *JAMA Neurology*.

The great news is that the results of vitamin D research are in practice. Dr. Cicero Galli Coimbra, a neurologist practicing in Sao Paulo, Brazil, has successfully treated MS patients with high-dose (40,000 to 200,000 IU) vitamin D on a daily basis. His Coimbra Protocol has successfully treated MS patients to the point where they are in complete remission!

"For a healthy person, I can say without a doubt that 10,000 IU of vitamin D a day will not pose any risk, quite the contrary. For those who suffer from any autoimmune disease, this dose will bring partial relief, but will not eliminate the problem. Higher doses can be used, provided this supplementation is done under medical supervision."

— Dr. Cicero Coimbra

Practice of the Coimbra Protocol has expanded beyond Brazil to other South American countries, Europe, the United States, and Canada. For more information about the Coimbra Protocol, its doctors and patients, please see my recommendations in the "Additional Resources" section near the back of this book.

Rheumatoid Arthritis (RA)

You most likely have seen countless commercial advertisements hawking remedies for arthritis, a disease for which there is no cure. Arthritis is the most common cause of disability in the United States, according to the Centers for Disease Control and Prevention.

Types of arthritis include rheumatoid arthritis and osteoarthritis. (Please see Chapter 12 for a discussion about vitamin D and osteoarthritis.)

Rheumatoid arthritis (RA) is an autoimmune disease that causes pain, swelling, and stiffness in the joints, mainly affecting the wrists, elbows, fingers, knees, ankles, toes, and neck. In RA patients the immune system attacks the joint lining, causing inflammation, usually striking both sides of the body at about the same time, resulting in severely impaired mobility in the upper or lower body.

Unlike the more common osteoarthritis, RA also can adversely affect the body's organ systems including the heart, lungs, kidneys, and nerves. Complications of RA can eventually destroy the joints as well as cause lung disease, heart failure, neuropathy, anemia, eye disease, or inflammation of the blood vessels.

About one percent of the global population suffers from RA. Between one and two million Americans suffer from RA. The majority of RA victims are women but men also develop the disease. Although the debilitating illness can occur at any age, RA usually strikes persons between the ages of 25 and 50.

A research team in India studied and compared the vitamin D levels of fifty rheumatoid arthritis patients with fifty healthy control subjects, all of whom were in the age group of 18-75 years. Eighty-four percent of RA patients were "vitamin D deficient" versus thirty-four percent of healthy control persons. Moreover, the lower the vitamin D levels in RA patients, the greater the disease activity. In other words, the vitamin D levels directly correlated with the intensity of the disease. Persons with RA who had higher vitamin D levels experienced less pain, swelling, and inflammation. The researchers concluded that "vitamin D deficiency is more common in RA patients and may be one of the *causes* leading to development or worsening of the disease." The study was published in a 2018 edition of the *Journal of Natural Science, Biology and Medicine*.

French researchers led a randomized, double-blind, placebo-controlled study that assessed the short-term effect of vitamin D for six months on rheumatoid arthritis patients. The research, published in a July 2018 issue of the journal *Clinical and Experimental Rheumatology*, indicated that six-month vitamin D supplementation in RA patients with vitamin D deficiency caused at least "a statistically significant improvement" in their functional disability.

Concluding Thoughts

Research evidence over the past few decades indicates a direct correlation between vitamin D levels and the incidence of autoimmune diseases. By reviewing the medical literature studying vitamin D and several, common autoimmune diseases, we see that most people who suffer from these conditions have low vitamin D levels. Furthermore, there is evidence to suggest that vitamin D supplementation at least during the early stages of autoimmunity may lessen the severity of the symptoms. I am encouraged by Dr. Coimbra's success in treating MS patients primarily with vitamin D, and hope that this practice could also treat other autoimmune diseases.

12

BONE DISEASES

As we age, major bone diseases might affect our quality of life including osteoarthritis and osteoporosis. Osteoarthritis is very painful. On the other hand, osteoporosis is silent until brittle bones break. Both chronic diseases are associated with deficiencies of vitamins D and K.

When we think about painful or frail bones, the mineral "calcium" most likely comes to mind. Calcium indeed is an important factor in bone health, but it does not act alone.

Vitamin D regulates the absorption of calcium and phosphorus in the intestines but needs vitamin K2 to move the calcium out of the bloodstream and soft tissues to the bones—where the calcium belongs.

Although I addressed vitamins D3 and K2, calcium, and phosphorus in the "Partners" chapter, I cannot overemphasize the importance of pairing D3 with K2 to strengthen your bones.

Osteoarthritis

Osteoarthritis (OA) is the most common form of arthritis and is the leading cause of chronic disability worldwide. In the United States, over 30 million people suffer from OA.

A progressive disease, OA is characterized by cartilage deterioration in joints, which results in bones rubbing together (bone-on-bone) that create pain, stiffness, and impaired movement. The disease usually affects the joints in the knees, hips, hands, feet, and spine.

Unfortunately, there is no cure for OA. However, scientific research has shown a possible preventative connection between vitamin D and OA:

- Researchers in China evaluated the effect of vitamin D in patients after knee or hip surgery by analyzing the results of twelve previous studies on the subject. The research team concluded in a 2018 edition of the *Annals of Nutrition and Metabolism* that the prevalence of vitamin D deficiency is high in patients who undergo knee or hip surgery. The Chinese team also indicated that low vitamin D "may affect the outcomes of orthopedic joint surgery." The clinical assessment of hip and knee surgery results, or scores, demonstrated significantly lower scores of patients who have vitamin D deficiency. Furthermore, post-operative patients stayed in the hospital at least one day longer than those who were vitamin-D-sufficient.

- In seeking to identify the cause of osteoarthritis, University of Creighton, Nebraska researchers reviewed medical literature to understand better the role of vitamin D in remodeling articular bone cartilage. While the researchers acknowledged that clinical trials have demonstrated that vitamin D deficiency poses an increased risk for OA, they stated that vitamin D supplementation's part in preventing or treating OA "remains uncertain." The study was published in a June 2017 issue of the *Orthopedic Journal of Sports Medicine*.

- An international research team studied the vitamin D blood levels of 418 participants who had knee OA. The team concluded that individuals who were low in vitamin D had an elevated risk of knee OA progression. In other words, OA most likely will get worse if vitamin D levels are low. The study was reported in the December 2014 issue of *The Journal of Nutrition*.

Osteoporosis

Osteoporosis is a common, loss-of-bone disease that can happen at any age, but it is prevalent in older adults. Globally, about one in three women over the age of 50, and one in five men older than 50 suffer from an osteoporotic fracture (usually in the wrists, hips, or spine) during their lifetime.

Osteoporosis essentially is a loss of bone mass and occurs when the body does not have the correct chemistry to strengthen bones. A condition called osteopenia, where bone density is lower than normal, can act as a precursor to osteoporosis. Both osteoporosis and osteopenia are silent medical conditions that are usually diagnosed when a bone fracture happens, although they can be diagnosed by a non-invasive, bone-density test called a DEXA (dual energy x-ray absorptiometry) scan. Persons over the age of 50 are usually encouraged by the medical community to undergo a periodic DEXA scan.

There is no identified cure for osteoporosis at the time of this writing. Nonetheless, some research has been conducted on the dynamic connection between osteoporosis and vitamins D and K:

- A European research team reviewed "evidence of the synergistic interplay between vitamins D and K on bone...health." The researchers concluded that the "current evidence supports the notion that joint supplementation of vitamins D and K might be more effective than the consumption of either alone for bone...health." This study was published in a 2017 issue of the *International Journal of Endocrinology.*

- The number of hip fractures in Norway's capital of Oslo ranks among the highest in the world. Researchers from the Oslo University Hospital examined the connection between vitamins K1 and D3 and an increased risk of hip fractures, comparing the blood levels of vitamin K1 and vitamin D3 with 111 hip fracture patients and 73 healthy controls. Discovering lower levels of vitamins K1 and D3 in the hip-fracture patients, the research team concluded that vitamin K1 and vitamin D3 are "independently and synergistically associated with the risk of hip fracture." The study was reported in the February 2015 issue of the journal *Clinical Nutrition.*

Concluding Thoughts

When I wrote this chapter, I had a dear friend in mind. Only in her fifties, she suffers from osteoarthritis in both hips, and needs hip replacements to relieve her pain and improve her quality of life. My heart goes out to her.

I cannot overemphasize the importance of supplementing jointly (no pun intended) with D3 and K2 daily to hopefully prevent or reduce the severity of debilitating bone diseases. The paucity of clinical trials testing the efficacy of these two nutrients is probably due to lack of funding. After all, most practices rely on prescribing pharmaceutical medications to prevent bone disease, rather than recommending supplements.

13

CANCER

Today a common perception is that cancer is almost inevitable because we are most likely genetically or environmentally disposed to developing some form of cancer during our lives. Our fears are not unfounded.

More than 8.2 million people worldwide annually perish from cancer. The United Nations' cancer research agency estimated that cancer will kill over 13.2 million people a year by 2030.

Cancer is the second most common cause of death in the United States. We should not acquiesce to cancer's death rate. Adequate vitamin D has the potential to prevent and treat different types of cancers. Let's look at how vitamin D works to prevent the development and growth of malignant cells.

The adult human body comprises about 100 trillion cells. Most of these cells include vitamin D receptors that receive, store, and, in some cases, produce activated vitamin D. Activated vitamin D influences cells to grow—and die—normally. When cells do not behave normally, they can proliferate and become "rogue" cells that offer an inviting home for cancer development. If the body has sufficient activated vitamin D stored in its cells, vitamin D will incite natural cell death, or apoptosis.

Vitamin D's capability to affect natural cell death negates the opportunity for cancer cells to proliferate, develop into a tumor, and spread to other parts of the body. This fact alone should encourage everyone to ensure their vitamin D levels are adequate!

Activated vitamin D's process of natural cell death holds great promise in the prevention and treatment of many types of cancer. The link between vitamin D and three prevalent types of cancer: breast, colorectal, and prostate is addressed in the next three chapters.

14

BREAST CANCER

We are simply inundated with the color pink during the month of October each year. Everywhere we look, we see various shades of pink to remind us that October is Breast Cancer Awareness Month.

Why, after over three decades of honoring annual Breast Cancer Awareness Month and billions of dollars poured into conventional research, does breast cancer remain the most common cancer among women in the world? Moreover, approximately 571,000 women around the globe are expected to die from breast cancer in 2018.

My years of delving into the medical literature suggest that we rise above the ubiquitous pink when we think about diagnosing and treating breast cancer. How about *preventing* breast cancer by reducing its risk with vitamin D? And how about increasing survival rates by *treating* breast cancer with safe, inexpensive, and non-invasive vitamin D supplementation?

Vitamin D May Prevent Breast Cancer

By attaining and maintaining adequate vitamin D levels in our bodies, we can potentially defend our lives against breast cancer. Breast (mammary gland) cells are replete with vitamin D receptors (VDR) that receive, store, and produce activated vitamin D. If these VDR are sufficiently active, they exude anti-cancer effects by: regulating cell differentiation, proliferation, and natural death (apoptosis) in breast tissue, as well as gene expression. If the VDR in breast tissues are not working at their optimal level, breast cancer may develop.

- A team of U.S. researchers investigated the association between vitamin levels and breast cancer risk across a wide range of vitamin D blood serum concentrations among women aged 55 and older. Published in a June 15, 2018 issue of the journal *PLOS One*, the study concluded that vitamin D levels of greater than or equal to 60 ng/mL, or 150 nmol/L, were most protective against the risk of breast cancer.

How Vitamin D May Treat Breast Cancer

Scientific evidence has proven that vitamin D receptors in breast tissue cells receive, store, and produce activated vitamin D. This fact alone indicates that vitamin D has the potential to treat breast cancer patients. Medical research also suggests that vitamin D may play a role in treating breast cancer.

- A U.S. study conducted by Kaiser Permanente Northern California investigated the vitamin D levels of 1,666 women who had been diagnosed with invasive breast cancer. The researchers stated that women with the highest vitamin D levels "had superior overall survival." The conclusions included "compelling observational evidence on the associations of vitamin D with lower risk of breast cancer morbidity and mortality." The research was published in the March 1, 2017 issue of *JAMA Oncology*.

- A study, led by the University of California San Diego (UCSD), offered a highly promising conclusion about the link between vitamin D and breast cancer mortality. After analyzing data from 4,443 breast cancer patients, the research team concluded that breast cancer patients who had an average vitamin D level of 30 ng/mL (75 nmol/L) were about twice as likely to survive the disease than women with levels averaging 17 ng/mL (42.5 nmol/L).

- The UCSD researchers also noted that the average vitamin D level in breast cancer patients in the United States is a paltry 17 ng/mL. Dr. Cedric Garland, a professor in UCSD's Department of Family and Preventive Medicine who participated in the study, suggested medical professionals consider adding vitamin D to breast cancer patients' standard care regimens. The study, published in a March 2014 edition of the journal *Anticancer Research*, concluded that "all patients with breast cancer" should have vitamin

D levels in the range of 30 to 80 ng/mL (75 to 200 nmol/L).

Adequate vitamin D supplementation in concert with alternative and integrative treatments may overcome breast cancer. If you have been diagnosed with breast cancer, you may want to consider vitamin D therapy by consulting your health care practitioner.

Concluding Thoughts

The American Cancer Society estimates that one in eight women in the United States will develop invasive breast cancer during their lifetime. In 2018, about 266,120 women in the United States will be diagnosed with invasive breast cancer. Why acquiesce to these statistics?

Vitamin D's capability to affect natural cell death and gene expression negates the opportunity for breast cancer cells to proliferate, develop into a tumor, and spread to other parts of the body. This fact alone should encourage everyone to ensure their vitamin D levels are adequate!

Compelling medical evidence supports the connection between vitamin D levels and the risk of developing breast cancer. High levels of vitamin D in the body directly correlate with a decreased risk of breast cancer. Furthermore, scientific studies suggest treating breast cancer with vitamin D supplementation. Vitamin D Wellness therapy is non-invasive, safe, and inexpensive.

15

COLORECTAL CANCER

Colorectal cancer (commonly called "colon cancer") is a silent killer that begins in the colon or rectum, which combined are referred to as the large intestine. According to a variety of sources, colorectal cancer is the third most common cancer in the United States as well as around the globe. The disease kills more than 50,000 people a year in the United States.

The risk for colorectal cancer over a lifetime is 1 in 22 in men, and 1 in 24 for women. The rate of colorectal cancer is decreasing, except among "younger people," a trend that prompted the American Cancer Society to recommend lowering the screening age from 50 to 45.

In the majority of people who acquire the disease, colorectal cancer develops slowly over several years with symptoms that can be interpreted as common complaints. Colorectal cancer usually develops as a non-cancerous polyp on the inner lining of the colon or rectum. Many polyps are benign but they can become cancerous as a result of inflammation.

Once cancer develops in a polyp, the cancer cells may eventually grow into the wall of the large intestine. Entry of cancer cells into the colon or rectum can facilitate metastasis: the spread of cancer to other organs, blood, or lymph nodes.

How Vitamin D Could Prevent Colorectal Cancer

Let's look at how adequate vitamin D status may play a significant role to stop colorectal cancer before it develops:

Over 95 percent of colorectal cancers—called adeno-carcinomas—begin in the colorectal mucosal cells that form mucus-producing glands to lubricate the lining of the colon and rectum. The mucosal cells also contain vitamin D receptors that receive and produce activated vitamin D.

Most medical experts agree that chronic inflammation can cause normal cells to go awry—hence, become cancerous. Not surprisingly, inflammatory bowel diseases including Crohn's disease and ulcerative colitis cause chronic inflammation of the colon. Once again, vitamin D's anti-inflammatory mechanisms help prevent inflammation—one of the initial conditions that could lead to the development of colorectal cancer.

- An international group of researchers from organizations including the American Cancer Society conducted a landmark study of vitamin D and colorectal cancer risk. The research team examined the data of over 12,000 participants to ascertain a vitamin D level that would decrease the risk of colorectal cancer. Published in the June 14, 2018 issue of the *Journal of Natural Cancer Institute*, the researchers concluded that higher vitamin D status (30-40 ng/mL or 75-100 nmol/L) is significantly associated with "substantially lower colorectal cancer risk."

How Vitamin D Could Treat Colorectal Cancer

We know that vitamin D receptors in the colon and rectum's mucosal cells both receive and produce activated vitamin D. This fact alone suggests that vitamin D has the potential to treat at least the early stages of colorectal cancer. However, at the time of this writing, there is little evidence to substantiate vitamin D as a treatment for colorectal cancer.

However, a study, conducted by Dana-Farber researchers, gives some hope that vitamin D supplementation may help treat colorectal cancer:

- At the January 12, 2015 meeting of the American Society of Cancer Oncology Gastrointestinal Cancers Symposium in San Francisco, a researcher presented the Dana-Farber team's findings about vitamin D's effect on metastatic colorectal patients. These patients had "high" vitamin D levels *before* chemotherapy and targeted-drug treatment. Patients who had the highest vitamin D levels survived on average 8.1 months longer than patients with the lowest levels.

- The study's lead author Kimmie Ng, MD, MPH, a medical oncologist at the Gastrointestinal Cancer Treatment Center at Dana-Farber, stated, "This is the largest study that has been undertaken of metastatic colorectal cancer patients and vitamin D. It's further supportive of the potential benefits of maintaining sufficient levels of vitamin D in improving patient survival times."

Concluding Thoughts

Adequate vitamin D status may significantly reduce the risk of developing colorectal cancer. Vitamin D status also may have the potential to treat colorectal cancer during its initial stages. Obviously, additional scientific research on humans needs to be done. Nonetheless, why risk getting this horrible cancer, when you can add vitamin D and its cofactors to your body to help prevent colorectal cancer?

16

PROSTATE CANCER

Prostate cancer is yet another silent but lethal cancer. Cancer of the prostate—a male reproductive gland—is the second-leading cause of cancer deaths of males in the United States. About 29,430 American men were expected to die of prostate cancer in 2018.

More than 164,000 new cases of prostate cancer arise each year in the United States. In the majority of men, the cancer develops slowly when the genes in the prostate cells change abnormally. The exact cause of prostate cancer remains unknown.

Age is a predominant risk factor for developing prostate cancer. About two out of every three cases are diagnosed in men over the age of 65. Prostate cancer is more common in African-American men than in males of other ethnicities. Another noteworthy statistic encompasses the geographic location of prostate cancer victims:

the disease is most common in North America and northwestern Europe.

Do these statistics ring a familiar bell? Let's see: people with darker skin color and living in higher latitudes have an increased risk of vitamin D deficiency. Adequate vitamin D status may play a significant role to stop prostate cancer before it begins. Evidence also suggests vitamin D may treat at least early stages of prostate cancer.

How Vitamin D Could Prevent Prostate Cancer

Prostate gland cells contain vitamin D receptors (VDR) that receive and produce activated vitamin D. If VDR are sufficiently active, they exude a number of anti-cancer effects including fighting inflammation and regulating gene expression to promote natural cell death. A sampling of medical studies supporting the connection between vitamin D and prostate cancer are:

- A study conducted in the United States examined the results of first-time prostate biopsies and compared them to the men's vitamin D levels. The researchers, from prestigious medical educational institutions in Chicago, Cleveland, and Philadelphia, found that the more aggressive tumors were linked to lower vitamin D levels. The research team also concluded: a) African-American males with low vitamin D levels had an increased risk of developing prostate cancer and b) European Americans and African-Americans men with both positive biopsies and low vitamin D levels had more advanced prostate cancer stages. The study was published in the May 1, 2014 issue of the journal *Clinical Cancer Research.*

How Vitamin D Could Treat Prostate Cancer

The VDR in prostate cells both receive and produce activated vitamin D. This fact alone suggests that vitamin D has the potential to treat at least the early stages of prostate cancer. Medical research suggests vitamin D may play a role in treating prostate cancer.

- Researchers in Paris, France looked at vitamin D as a treatment for men with low-risk prostate cancer. Their findings, published on May 15, 2018 in *Nature Reviews Urology,* suggested that vitamin D may prevent the progression of early-stage prostate tumors.

- Six U.S. researchers investigated vitamin D's connection to survival from prostate cancer by studying military veterans who had prostate cancer. The scientists found that low vitamin D status is associated with a decreased likelihood after being diagnosed with prostate cancer. The research team recommended vitamin D supplementation in veterans with prostate cancer. The study was published in the January 2014 issue of *Military Medicine.*

Concluding Thoughts

Adequate vitamin D status may significantly reduce the risk of developing prostate cancer. Healthy vitamin D status also may have the potential to treat prostate cancer at least during its initial stages. Guys, why risk getting this potentially deadly cancer?

17

CARDIOVASCULAR DISEASE

Cardiovascular disease (CVD) is the *leading global cause of death* with more than 17.9 million deaths in 2015. This number is predicted to increase to 23.6 million deaths by 2030.

About one in every three Americans succumbs to CVD. According to a 2018 American Heart Association (AHA) statistical report, every 38 seconds, someone in the United States dies from a heart-related event.

CVD comprises any medical condition affecting the heart and arteries. Examples of CVD include: high blood pressure (hypertension); peripheral arterial disease; blocked arteries (coronary heart disease); stroke; heart attack (myocardial infarction); chest pain (angina); hardening of the arteries (atherosclerosis); blood clotting (thrombosis); inflammatory heart diseases; and vein inflammation (phlebitis). High blood pressure, the most common CVD in the United States, is often a prelude to more serious CVD such as coronary heart disease, atherosclerosis, stroke, and heart attack.

Heart disease is the No. 1 killer of American females. Not surprisingly, diagnosis of some CVD types is more difficult in women than men. Females are more likely to develop a CVD at a less detectable level—in tiny micro-vessels—than men, who tend to get blockages in the larger blood vessels of the heart. About fifty percent of women do not experience chest pain, the most apparent CVD symptom in men. Other CVD warning signs include: shortness of breath; persistent, unexplainable fatigue; indigestion; nausea; arm pain (especially in the left arm); and jaw or throat pain.

Who is at Risk to Develop CVD?

The majority of Americans adults are at risk to develop at least one type of CVD. Lifestyle choices contribute to a higher risk of developing CVD as well as specific medical conditions. Nine out of ten heart disease patients have at least one risk factor. According to the AHA, these risk factors include: high blood pressure (a CVD that can cause other CVDs); high cholesterol; diabetes; chronic kidney disease; unhealthy diet; smoking; alcohol use; overweight-ness and obesity; and physical inactivity.

The risk of developing CVD is not all about disease and lifestyle. Another CVD risk factor is vitamin D deficiency.

Vitamin D's powerful functions may decrease the risk of developing CVD. The cardiovascular system hosts vitamin D in a big way. The heart muscle cells and the blood vessels' smooth muscle cells contain the key enzyme that converts circulating vitamin D to activated vitamin D.

Vitamin D receptors (VDR) reside in the heart muscle cells, the arteries, the smooth muscle cells in the blood vessel walls, and the lining of the blood vessels (endothelium). The omnipresence of VDR in the cardiovascular system may result in activated vitamin D that promotes heart and vascular health by minimizing plaque development, reducing inflammation, and enhancing muscle strength.

- Vitamins D and K clean the heart and blood vessels by moving calcium to your bones and teeth rather than to cardiovascular tissues. Adequate vitamins D and K may prevent CVDs exacerbated by calcium deposits that form plaque: hardening of the arteries (atherosclerosis); peripheral artery disease; coronary heart disease; and blood clotting (thrombosis).

- Vitamin D's anti-inflammatory properties fight viruses and bacteria. Adequate vitamin D levels may reduce inflammatory heart diseases such as myocarditis, pericarditis, and endocarditis. Phlebitis, or vein inflammation, is another type of CVD that may be prevented by vitamin D.

- Activated vitamin D maintains and strengthens the heart muscle and artery muscle cells. The heart comprises mostly muscle so a weak heart can lead to a host of serious conditions including heart failure.

A European research team reviewed "evidence of the synergistic interplay between vitamins D and K on… cardiovascular health." The researchers concluded that the "current evidence supports the notion that joint supplementation of vitamins D and K might be more effective than the consumption of either alone for … cardiovascular health." This study was published in a 2017 issue of the *International Journal of Endocrinology*.

How Can Vitamin D Treat CVD?

To the best of my knowledge, few studies examining vitamin D's role in treatment of CVDs have been conducted at the time of this writing. However, I am encouraged by Ohio University in Athens, Ohio research on the effect of vitamin D on the endothelium. The lining of the entire circulatory system acts more like an organ, and damage to it, such as high blood pressure and atherosclerosis, may be repaired by adequate vitamin D.

- Using nanosensors to measure the impact of activated vitamin D on molecular mechanisms in damaged human endothelial cells, the researchers, led by Professor Tadeusz Malinski, surmised that vitamin D may play a key role in preserving endothelium as well as repairing damaged endothelium. Dr. Malinski cautioned that although many heart attack patients have a vitamin D deficiency, "It doesn't mean that the deficiency caused the heart attack but it increased the risk of heart attack." This study was published in the January 19, 2018 issue of *the International Journal of Nanomedicine*.

Concluding Thoughts

Sufficient vitamin D supplementation may combat CVDs. Vitamin D's functions, including working with vitamin K to move calcium to the bones and teeth; fighting bacteria and viruses; and strengthening heart and arterial muscles, play an important role in cardiovascular health.

Observational studies indicate that persons with higher circulating vitamin D enjoy a lower risk of developing or dying from CVDs. We await randomized controlled trials that either demonstrate or disprove that adequate vitamin D lowers the incidences of CVDs.

Writing this chapter resonated personally with me. In November 2018, my dear brother-in-law Michael, who was only 50, suddenly died from massive heart failure. Our family found a signed copy of Defend Your Life *(my first book) in a place of prominence on his coffee table. Did he read about vitamin D benefits and cardiovascular disease? I will never know but he had not consulted a medical doctor in over twenty years. I can only think of how a CT cardiac calcium (CAC) scoring test (discussed in Chapter 4) may have saved his young, vibrant life.*

PART IV

Vitamin D Wellness

18

VITAMIN D WELLNESS PROTOCOL

Vitamin D is essential to our health and quality of life. Virtually every cell in our body contains a vitamin D receptor (VDR). When a VDR is activated by a sufficient intake of vitamin D, good things happen. Vitamin D's mechanisms of action include: anti-microbial, anti-cancer, anti-inflammatory. In other words, scientific research indicates that vitamin D deficiency is connected to a wide array of serious medical conditions such as cancer, cardiovascular disease, depression, as well as multiple sclerosis and other autoimmune diseases.

Due to our modern lifestyles and conventional medical practices, we tend to get little vitamin D from its natural source, the ultraviolet B (UVB) rays of the sun. From living, commuting, and working indoors to fretfully slapping sunscreen all over our skin, we appear intent on denying ourselves this essential nutrient. As the majority of diets are severely lacking in vitamin D, the most practical way of getting adequate vitamin D is by taking an inexpensive daily, oral D3 supplement.

As someone who is impassioned with the health benefits of vitamin D, my vitamin D level has been optimal (more than 100 ng/mL) for years, despite my inherited VDR gene variants. Anyone who has one or more VDR gene variants can overcome this defect by raising one's levels to at least 100 ng/mL (250 nmol/L). In fact, by following my three-nutrient protocol you may overcome any vitamin D-related genetic disposition within weeks or a few months.

The Vitamin D Wellness Protocol

More than 50,000 people have accessed the three-nutrient, Vitamin D Wellness Protocol on my website: smilinsuepubs.com. Here is the Protocol in a nutshell:

Vitamin D: Most diets do not contain adequate vitamin D3. Start by taking 5,000 IU *daily* of vitamin D3 oil-based (soft gels or liquid) supplements with or right after your breakfast. After the first week, take 10,000 IU a day. Enjoy direct noon sun exposure for up to 15-20 minutes a day, when possible.

Vitamin K2: A vitamin K2 diet includes lots of grass-fed meat and dairy products. Since most of us are lacking a daily, abundant intake of grass-fed foods, supplement with about 100 mcg of vitamin K2 (MK-7). Take your K2 and D3 together with, or right after your breakfast that includes healthy fats such as egg yolks, cottage cheese, other cheeses, avocado, and nuts. NOTE: 1) *Please do not take any form of vitamin K if you are on blood-thinning medication without the approval of your health care practitioner.* 2) If you are taking thyroid medication, please avoid taking a soy-based (natto) vitamin K2 MK-7. Soy may disrupt the efficacy of thyroid hormone medication.

Magnesium: Magnesium-rich foods include leafy green vegetables such as spinach, legumes, avocado, nuts, seeds, and dark chocolates. A *daily* supplement of magnesium glycinate (or magnesium malate if you do not have access to magnesium glycinate) of 400 to 600 mg should boost your levels of this essential mineral. Take your magnesium glycinate before bedtime as the glycine in this supplement has a calming effect that should foster sleep. On the other hand, magnesium malate should be taken in the morning as it fosters energy.

From assisting thousands of members of the Vitamin D Wellness support group on Facebook, our team has found that some people have difficulty swallowing or ingesting magnesium capsules. If you are one of those individuals, you can open the capsules and sprinkle the magnesium contents into foods such as applesauce. Or you could consume *daily* foods replete with magnesium that are listed in the above paragraph. As amounts of these foods vary from individual-to-individual, we suggest you check online for food quantities commensurate with your needs.

PLEASE NOTE: Persons taking thyroid medication should wait at least *four* hours before taking any magnesium or other mineral supplements.

Specific brands of vitamins D3 and K2 MK-7, and magnesium are listed (and linked) in the online Protocol via smilinsuepubs.com. Suggested supplements for children are also included.

Concluding Thoughts

Well, there you have it! An insightful look at vitamin D, its partners, as well as medical and scientific research. This chapter offers a culmination of my efforts: the easy-to-follow Vitamin D Wellness Protocol. I wish you much success with improved health!

ADDITIONAL VITAMIN D RESOURCES

Autism

Book: *Autism Causes: Prevention and Treatment* by John J. Cannell. 2015. Paper and electronic copies are available via Amazon.

Video: *The Connection between Vitamin D and Autism* by Susan Rex Ryan. YouTube. May 23, 2015 presentation to the Autism One conference in Chicago.

Depression and Methylation (including VDR) Genetics

Book: *Silent Inheritance: Are You Predisposed to Depression?* by Susan Rex Ryan. 2017. Paper and electronic copies are available via Amazon.

Multiple Sclerosis and other Autoimmune Diseases

Book: *Multiple Sclerosis and (lots of) Vitamin D: My Eight-Year Treatment with The Coimbra Protocol for Autoimmune Diseases* by Ana Claudia Domene. 2016. Paper and electronic copies are available via Amazon.

Website: www.CoimbraProtocol 'dot' com. Lots of information on the Coimbra Protocol and the doctors who treat patients with it.

Sunlight

Book: *Embrace the Sun: Are You Dying in the Dark?* By Marc B. Sorenson and William B. Grant. 2018. Paper copy is available via Amazon.

Vitamin D and Other Health Topics

Website: www.smilinsuepubs 'dot' com. The author's website and blog.

Website: www.vitaminDcouncil 'dot' org. Dr. Cannell's vitamin D non-profit.

Website: www.grassrootshealth 'dot' net. Vitamin D-related information.

BIBLIOGRAPHY

Abreo, A et al. "The impact of a modifiable risk factor reduction on childhood asthma development." *Clinical and Translational Medicine.* 2018 Jun 11;7(1):15.

Al-Ajlan, A et al. "Lower vitamin D levels in Saudi pregnant women are associated with higher risk of GDM." *BMC Pregnancy & Childbirth.* 2018 Apr 10;18(1):86.

Alansari, K et al. "Rapid vs Maintenance Vitamin D Supplementation in Deficient Children with Asthma to Prevent Exacerbations." *Chest.* 2017 Sep;152(3):527-536.

Ali, AM et al. "Effect of alfacalcidol on the pulmonary function of adult asthmatic patients: A randomized trial." *Annals of Allergy, Asthma & Immunology.* 2017 May;118(5):557-563.

Allan, KM et al. "Maternal vitamins D and E intakes during pregnancy are associated with asthma in children." *European Respiratory Journal.* 2015 Apr; 45(4):1027-36.

American Society of Anesthesiologists. "Moms-to-be with low vitamin D levels could have more painful labors." *Science Daily.* 2014 Oct 14.

Annweiler, C et al. "Vitamin D and cognition in older adults: updated international recommendations." *Journal of Internal Medicine.* 2015 Jan;277(1):45-57.

Bakr, HG and Meawed, TE. "Relevance of 25(OH) Vitamin D deficiency on Hashimoto's Thyroiditis. *Egyptian Journal of Immunology.* 2017 Jun;24(2):53-62.

Butts, S et al. "Vitamin D may be key for pregnant women with polycystic ovary syndrome." *Science Daily.* 2017 Nov 6.

Cannell, John J. *Autism Causes: Prevention and Treatment.* Sunrise River Press. 2015.

Capiod, T et al. "Do dietary calcium and vitamin D matter in men with prostate cancer?" *Nature Reviews Urology.* 2018 May 15.

Chrisostomo, KR et al. "The prevalence and clinical associations of hypovitaminosis D in pregnant women from Brazil." *International Journal of Gynecology & Obstetrics.* 2018 Jan 26.

Der, T et al. "Vitamin D and prostate cancer survival in veterans." *Military Medicine.* 2014 Jan;179(1):81-84.

Feart, C et al. "Associations of lower vitamin D concentrations with cognitive decline and long-term risk of dementia and Alzheimer's disease in older adults." *Alzheimer's & Dementia.* 2017 Nov;13(11):1207-1216.

Garfinkel, RJ et al. "Vitamin D and Its Effects on Articular Cartilage and Osteoarthritis." *Orthopedic Journal of Sports Medicine.* 2017 Jun 20;5(6).

Goncalves, DR et al. "Recurrent pregnancy loss and vitamin D: A review of the literature." *American Journal of Reproductive Immunology.* 2018 Jul 27:e13022.

Goodwill, AM et al. "Vitamin D status is associated with executive function a decade later: Data from the Women's Healthy Ageing Project." *Maturitas.* 2018 Jan;107:56-62.

Grundy, SM et al. "Guideline on Management of Blood Cholesterol: A Report of the American College of Cardiology/American Heart Association Task Force on Clinical Practice Guidelines." *Journal of the American College of Cardiology.* 2018 Nov 8.

Harvey, NC et al. "Maternal antenatal vitamin D status and offspring muscle development: findings from the Southampton Women's Survey." *Journal of Clinical Endocrinology and Metabolism.* 2014 Jan;99(1):330-7.

Heyden EL and Wimalawansa SJ. "Vitamin D: Effects on human reproduction, pregnancy, and fetal well-being." *Journal of Biochemistry and Molecular Biology.* 2018 Jun;180:41-50.

Hollis, BW et al. "Maternal Versus Infant Vitamin D Supplementation During Lactation: A Randomized Controlled Trial." *Pediatrics.* 2015 Oct;136(4):625-34.

Jia, F et al. "Fluctuations in clinical symptoms with changes in serum 25(OH) vitamin D levels in autistic children: Three case report." *Nutritional Neuroscience.* 2018 Apr 8:1-4.

Khan, A et al."Nanomedical studies of the restoration of nitric oxide/ peroxynitrite balance in dysfunctional endothelium by 1,25-dihydroxyvitamin D3—clinical applications for cardiovascular diseases." *International Journal of Nanomedicine.* 2018 Jan 19;13:455-466.

Licher, S et al. "Vitamin D and the Risk of Dementia: The Rotterdam Study." *Journal of Alzheimer's Disease.* 2017;60(3):989-997.

Lukaszyk, E et al. "Cognitive Functioning of Geriatric Patients: Is Hypovitaminosis D the Next Marker of Cognitive Dysfunction and Dementia?" *Nutrients.* 2018 Aug 16;10(80).

Mak, A. "The Impact of Vitamin D on the Immunopathophysiology, Disease Activity, and Extra-Musculoskeletal Manifestations of Systemic Lupus Erythematosus." *International Journal of Molecular Sciences.* 2018 Aug 10;19(8).

Martineau, AR et al. "Vitamin D supplementation to prevent acute respiratory tract infections: systematic review and meta-analysis of individual participant data." *British Medical Journal.* 2017 Feb 15:356:i6583.

McCullough, ML et al. "Circulating Vitamin D and Colorectal Cancer Risk: An International Pooling Project of 17 Cohorts." *Journal of the National Cancer Institute.* 2018 Jun 14.

McCullough, PJ et al. "Daily oral dosing of vitamin D3 using 5,000 to 50,000 international units a day in long-term hospitalized patients: Insights from a seven year experience." *Journal of Steroid Biochemistry and Molecular Biology.* 2019 Jan 3.

McDonnell, SL et al. "Breast cancer risk markedly lower with serum 25-hydroxyvitamin D concentrations greater or equal to 60 vs less than 20 ng/mL (150 vs 50 nmol/L): Pooled analysis of two randomized trials and a prospective cohort." *PLOS One.* 2018 Jun 15;13(6) e0199265.

McDonnell, SL et al. "Maternal 25(OH)D concentrations greater than or equal to 40 ng/mL associated with 60% lower preterm birth risk among general obstetrical patients at an urban medical center." *PLOS One.* 2017 Jul 24:12(7) e0180483.

McLaughlin, L et al. "Vitamin D for the treatment of multiple sclerosis: a meta-analysis." *Journal of Neurology.* 2018 Dec;265(12):2893-2905.

Meena, N et al. "Assessment of Vitamin D in Rheumatoid Arthritis and Its correlation with Disease Activity." *Journal of Natural Science, Biology and Medicine.* 2018 Jan-Jun;9(1):54-58.

Mumford, SL et al. "Association of preconception serum 25-hydroxyvitamin D concentrations with livebirth and pregnancy loss: a prospective cohort study." *The Lancet Diabetes & Endoctinology.* 2018 Sep;6(9):725-732.

Murphy, AB et al. "Vitamin D deficiency predicts prostate biopsy outcomes." *Clinical Cancer Research.* 2014 May 1;20(9):2289-99.

Muscogiuri, G et al. "Shedding new light on female fertility: The role of vitamin D." *Review of Endocrinology & Metabolism Disorders.* 2017 Sep:18(3);273-283.

Ng, Kimmie. "New study shows high vitamin D levels increase survival of patients with metastatic colorectal cancer." *Dana-Farber Cancer Institute.* 2015 Jan 12.

Nielsen, NM et al. "Neonatal vitamin D status and risk of multiple sclerosis: A population-based case-control study." *Neurology.* 2017 Jan 3;88(1):44-51.

Niruban, SJ et al. "Association between vitamin D and respiratory outcomes in Canadian adolescents and adults." *Journal of Asthma.* 2015 Sep;52(7):653-61.

Norris, JM et al. "Plasma 25-Hydroxyvitamin D Concentration and Risk of Islet Autoimmunity." *Diabetes.* 2018 Jan;67(1):146-154.

Obermer, Edgar. "Vitamin-D Requirements in Pregnancy." *British Medical Journal.* 1947.

Omotobara-Yabe, T et al. "Vitamin D deficiency associated with dilated cardiomyopathy in early infancy caused by maternal cholestasis." *Clinical Pediatric Endocrinology.* 2018;27(3):187-192.

Patrick, RP and Ames, BN. "Vitamin D hormone regulates serotonin synthesis. Part 1: relevance for autism." *FASEB Journal.* 2014 Jun;28(6):2398-413.

Pfotenhauer, KM and Shubrook, JH. "Vitamin D Deficiency, its Role in Health and Disease, and Current Supplementation Recommendations." *The Journal of American Osteopathic Association.* 2017 May 1;117(5):301-305.

Rajan, KB et al. "Cognitive impairment 18 years before clinical diagnosis of Alzheimer disease dementia." *Neurology.* 2015 Sep 8;85(10):898-904.

Saad, K et al. "Vitamin D status in autism spectrum disorders and the efficacy vitamin D supplementation in autistic children." *Nutritional Neuroscience.* 2016 Oct;19(8):346-351.

Serrano-Diaz, NC et al. "Vitamin D and risk of preeclampsia: A systematic review and meta-analysis." *Biomedical.* 2018 May 1;38 Suppl 1:43-53.

Solidoro, P et al. "Asthmatic Patients with Vitamin D Deficiency have Decreased Exacerbations after Vitamin Replacement." *Nutrients.* 2017 Nov 11;9(11).

Soubrier, M et al. "A randomized, double-blind, placebo-controlled study assessing the efficacy of high doses of vitamin D on functional disability in patients with rheumatoid arthritis." *Clinical and Experimental Rheumatology.* 2018 Jul 18.

Thandrayen, K and Pettifor, JM. "The roles of vitamin D and dietary calcium in nutritional rickets." *Bone Reports.* 2018 Jan 31;8:81-89.

Tobergsen, AC et al. "Vitamin K1 and 25(OH)D are independently and synergistically associated with a risk of a hip fracture in an elderly population: a case control study." *Clinical Nutrition.* 2015 Feb;34(1):101-6.

Van Ballegooijen, AJ et al. "The Synergistic Interplay between Vitamins D and K for Bone and Cardiovascular Health: A Narrative Review." *International Journal of Endocrinology.* 2017;2017:7454376.

Wang, C et al. "Correlation between neonatal vitamin D level & maternal vitamin D level." *Chinese Journal of Contemporary Pediatrics.* 2016 Jan;18(1):20-3.

Weernink, MG et al. "Insufficient vitamin D supplement use during pregnancy and early childhood: a risk factor for positional skull deformation." *Maternal & Childhood Nutrition.* 2016 Jan;12(1):177-88.

Wilson, RL et al. "Vitamin D levels in Australian and New Zealand cohort and the association with pregnancy outcomes." *BMC Pregnancy & Childbirth.* 2018 Jun 20;18(1):251.

Wu, DM et al. "Relationship between Neonatal Vitamin D at Birth and Risk of Autism Spectrum Disorders: the NBSIB Study." *Journal of Bone and Mineral Research.* 2018 Mar;33(3):458-466.

Yao, S et al. "Association of Serum Level of Vitamin D at Diagnosis with Breast Cancer Survival: A Case-Cohort Analysis in the Pathways Study." *JAMA Oncology.* 2017 Mar 1;3(3):351-357.

Zhang, FF et al. "Vitamin D Deficiency is associated with progression of knee osteoarthritis." *The Journal of Nutrition.* 2014 Dec;144(12):2002-08.

Zhang, G et al. "Effects of vitamin D on apoptosis of T-lymphocyte subsets in neonatal sepsis." *Experimental and Therapeutic Medicine.* 2018 Aug;16(2):629-634.

Zhang, H et al. "Vitamin D status and Patient Outcomes after Knee and Hip Surgery: A Meta-Analysis." *Annals of Nutrition and Metabolism.* 2018;73(2):121-130.

Index

ACKNOWLEDGMENTS

Defend Your Life II would not exist without the wonderful research that has been published on vitamin D and its potential health benefits. I thank the dozens of researchers and scientists who are as passionate about exploring vitamin D's role in human health as I am.

Thank you to the people who lead non-profit organizations that educate the public about vitamin D. These fine folks include John J. Cannell, MD, founder of the Vitamin D Council; Carole Baggerly of Grassroots Health; and Perry Holman of Canada's Vitamin D Society.

Special thanks to a dear friend who reviewed my draft work to make it better for you, the reader.

The cover of Defend Your Life II is a product of a superb graphic design professional named Shannon Bodie of BookWise Design in Oregon. The visual magic created by Shannon and her team enhances the positive vibes of this book.

Tons of gratitude to the administrators of the Vitamin D Wellness support group on Facebook. The admin team tirelessly responds to daily questions and offers lots of supports to our thousands of Vitamin D Wellness members.

Finally, thank you to my wonderful husband, Dave, my friends, and my great families: the Rexes and the Ryans. I am blessed with the best.

ABOUT THE AUTHOR

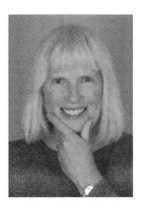

Susan "Sue" Rex Ryan was born and raised in the Philadelphia, Pennsylvania area. She earned a Bachelor of Science degree at Georgetown University, concentrating on languages and linguistics. Sue also holds a Master of Science degree from the U.S. military's National War College in Washington, D.C. In addition, she has earned scores of Continuing Medical Education (CME) credits from accredited U.S. medical programs approved by, inter alia, The American Academy of Family Physicians.

Her first book entitled *Defend Your Life* discusses the many health benefits of vitamin D and has garnered global accolades as an Amazon bestseller. In addition, *Defend Your Life* won a prestigious Mom's Choice Award®, an international awards program that recognizes authors and others for their efforts in creating quality family-friendly media products.

In 2015, Sue founded a private vitamin D support group in social media that has thousands of members. She also established her three-nutrient Vitamin D Protocol that has helped thousands enjoy better health.

By communicating with members from around the world, she learned that many endure methylation issues that adversely affect their brain health. By connecting the dots with medical literature research and her own experiences, Sue wrote her second book, entitled *Silent Inheritance* and published in November 2017.

Sue and her husband Dave reside in the sunny suburbs of beautiful Las Vegas, Nevada. They enjoy traveling to visit family and friends, as well as experiencing life in far-flung locations including Sri Lanka, Easter Island, and French Polynesia.

Follow Sue's commentary on Twitter @vitD3Sue. She welcomes your visit to her website smilinsuepubs.com that is replete with her blog articles about health topics.